# Frontiers in Anti-Infective Agents

## *(Volume 6)*

### Edited by

**Parvesh Singh**
*School of Chemistry and Physics*
*University of Kwa-Zulu Natal (UKZN)*
*Westville Campus, Durban*
*South Africa*

**Vipan Kumar**
*Department of Chemistry*
*Guru Nanak Dev University*
*Amritsar*
*India*

&

**Rajshekhar Karpoormath**
*Department of Pharmaceutical Chemistry*
*University of Kwa-Zulu Natal (UKZN)*
*Westville Campus, Durban*
*South Africa*

# Frontiers in Anti-Infective Agents

*Volume # 6*

Editors: Parvesh Singh, Vipan Kumar and Rajshekhar Karpoormath

ISSN (Online): 2705-1080

ISSN (Print): 2705-1072

ISBN (Online): 978-981-4998-42-0

ISBN (Print): 978-981-4998-43-7

ISBN (Paperback): 978-981-4998-44-4

need for a court order if at any point you breach any terms of this License Agreement. In no event will any delay or failure by Bentham Science Publishers in enforcing your compliance with this License Agreement constitute a waiver of any of its rights.

3. You acknowledge that you have read this License Agreement, and agree to be bound by its terms and conditions. To the extent that any other terms and conditions presented on any website of Bentham Science Publishers conflict with, or are inconsistent with, the terms and conditions set out in this License Agreement, you acknowledge that the terms and conditions set out in this License Agreement shall prevail.

**Bentham Science Publishers Pte. Ltd.**
80 Robinson Road #02-00
Singapore 068898
Singapore
Email: subscriptions@benthamscience.net

**BENTHAM SCIENCE**

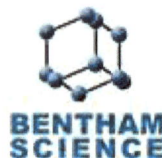

# CONTENTS

# PREFACE

Pathogens have historically affected human populations worldwide, resulting in epidemics and pandemics of different origins and epidemiology, as well as high mortality rates. Despite advancements in detection mechanisms and treatment of many known diseases through the development of novel drugs, the increase in the pace of evolution of drug resistance remains the greatest obstacle in drug design and discovery. The most recent threat to mankind is the SARS-coronavirus-2 (COVID-19), a viral zoonosis, which is difficult to diagnose due to many symptomatic similarities to influenza. Approaching the virus *via* a standardised treatment protocol has been inefficacious due to its rapid mutation, either being more virulent or becoming drug-resistant. The viral infection has engulfed the world in a fight response, in search of an appropriate vaccine or treatment to reduce the risk of infection and loss of human life. Biomolecular engineering and molecular bio-computing have been our greatest tools in drug discovery and development. It has enabled the repurposing of existing drugs by understanding the structure-activity relationship and pharmacokinetic properties against new targets or biological systems.

The book offers an insightful perspective on the most up-to-date developments and research engaged in the combat against pathogens and COVID-19. The contributions from distinguished researchers and leaders in their field are a critical analysis of vaccine development strategies, novel heterocyclic drug scaffolds, the history and biology of infection, and natural products as quorum sensors.

The chapter by Arindam Mitra emphasises reverse vaccinology approaches in vaccine design, intuitively targeting multiple pathogens, including the novel coronavirus, to combat the current pandemic of COVID-19. It also highlights the major advantages of reverse vaccinology for the discovery of novel vaccines with reduced time and cost in development. The second chapter by N. Ramalakshmi *et al.* is a critical review of leptospirosis and its treatment. The current remedies for milder cases of leptospirosis involve antibiotic administration *viz* penicillin, ampicillin, cefmetazole, oxalactam, ceftizoxime, and cefotaxime. This review summarizes the most recent literature on synthetic lead molecules, natural product chemotherapies, and drug targets. The third chapter by Nachimuthu Ramesh *et al.* sheds light on phage therapy and its evolution from lab to bedside endpoints in treating patients. The history and fundamentals of phage biology and its significance in treating infectious diseases have been provided, with commercialization strategies undertaken by the pharmaceutical industry. The fourth chapter by Debaprasad Parai *et al.* focuses on quorum sensing inhibitors (QSIs) from natural products. Quorum sensing is a signalling process, which regulates the expression of several virulence factors in both gram-negative and gram-positive bacteria *via* an autoinducing loop. When a critical bacterial cell density is reached, a complex of regulatory proteins and specific signalling molecules enable the autoinduction of the quorum sensor and the expression of the target genes. This chapter provides a literature review describing the various QSIs obtained from natural sources and their role as anti-infective agents. The fifth chapter by Shaik Baji Baba *et al.* reveals the importance of nitrogen and oxygen-based heterocycles as potential anti-infective agents. It details the development of 1,2,4-triazoles, isatin, and coumarin-based anti-infective agents. Structure-activity relationship studies provide scope for future researchers to develop the most effective and least toxic anti-infective agents.

We would like to acknowledge the expert contributions of the authors mentioned in the review articles in accomplishing this book, which forms an updated base platform for novel drug discovery and development against infective agents. Each author has been recognised as a dynamic leader in their field and we wish them well for their future research. We reserve a special recognition for the Bentham Science Publishing team, particularly Mrs. Fariya Zulfiqar (Manager Publications) and Mr. Mahmood Alam (Editorial Director), for the timely production of the 6ᵗʰ volume and promotion of this scientific collaboration.

**Parvesh Singh**
School of Chemistry and Physics
University of Kwa-Zulu Natal (UKZN)
Westville campus, Durban
South Africa

**Vipan Kumar**
Department of Chemistry
Guru Nanak Dev University
Amritsar
India

&

**Rajshekhar Karpoormath**
Department of Pharmaceutical Chemistry
University of Kwa-Zulu Natal (UKZN)
Westville Campus, Durban
South Africa

# List of Contributors

**A. Puratchikody**  University College of Engineering, Bharathidasan Institute of Technology Campus, Anna University, Tiruchirappalli, India

**Archana Loganathan**  Antibiotic Resistance and Phage Therapy Laboratory, School of Bio Sciences and Technology, Vellore Institute of Technology, Vellore, India

**Arindam Mitra**  Department of Microbiology, School of Life Science and Biotechnology, Adamas University, Kolkata, India

**Debaprasad Parai**  Department of Microbiology, University of Kalyani, Kalyani, West Bengal, India

**Kandasamy Eniyan**  Antibiotic Resistance and Phage Therapy Laboratory, School of Bio Sciences and Technology, Vellore Institute of Technology, Vellore, India

**N. Ramalakshmi**  C.L Baid Metha College of Pharmacy, Chennai, India

**Nachimuthu Ramesh**  Antibiotic Resistance and Phage Therapy Laboratory, School of Bio Sciences and Technology, Vellore Institute of Technology, Vellore, India

**Naresh Kumar Katari**  School of Chemistry & Physics, College of Agriculture, Engineering & Science, Westville Campus, University of KwaZulu-Natal, P Bag X 54001, Durban-4000, South Africa
Department of Chemistry, School of Science, GITAM Deemed to be University, Hyderabad, Telangana 502329,, India

**Pia Dey**  Department of Microbiology, University of Kalyani, WB, India- 741235

**Prasanth Manohar**  Zhejiang University-University of Edinburgh (ZJU-UoE) Institute, Zhejiang University, Haining, Zhejiang, P.R.China and The Second Affiliated Hospital Zhejiang University (SAHZU), School of Medicine, Hangzhou, P.R.China

**Rambabu Gundla**  School of Chemistry & Physics, College of Agriculture, Engineering & Science, Westville Campus, University of KwaZulu-Natal, P Bag X 54001, Durban-4000, South Africa

**S. Arunkumar**  SRM Modinagar College of Pharmacy, Modinagar, India

**Samir Kumar Mukherjee**  Department of Microbiology, University of Kalyani, Kalyani, West Bengal, India

**Sebastian Leptihn**  Antibiotic Resistance and Phage Therapy Laboratory, School of Bio Sciences and Technology, Vellore Institute of Technology, Vellore, India
Department of Infectious Diseases, Sir Run Run Shaw Hospital, Zhejiang University School of Medicine, Hangzhou, P.R. China
Infection Medicine, Biomedical Sciences, Edinburgh Medical School, College of Medicine and Veterinary Medicine, The University of Edinburgh, 1 George Square, Edinburgh, EH8 9JZ, United Kingdom

**Shaik Baji Baba**  School of Chemistry & Physics, College of Agriculture, Engineering & Science, Westville Campus, University of KwaZulu-Natal, P Bag X 54001, Durban-4000, South Africa

# CHAPTER 1

# Reverse Vaccinology Approaches for Rapid Vaccine Design Against Emerging Infectious Diseases

**Arindam Mitra**[1,*]

[1] *Department of Microbiology, School of Life Science and Biotechnology, Adamas University, Kolkata, India*

**Abstract:** Reverse vaccinology uses computational approaches to identify potential vaccine candidates. With the increasing pace of genome sequencing, it is possible to identify all potential antigens from any sequenced pathogen. Reverse vaccinology uses computational data to identify potential antigens, express those potential antigens, and then screen them further for protective immune response. Thus, reverse vaccinology offers several advantages and enables identifying novel antigens even if the expression level is low or not abundant. Besides, reverse vaccinology approaches offer reduced time and reduced cost for the development of vaccines compared to conventional vaccination methods. Such a timely, speedy, and economical process for developing vaccines without compromising safety and immunogenicity is the urgent need of the hour to combat many emerging pathogens, including SARS-CoV-2. This chapter summarizes approaches and challenges in developing vaccines against many emerging pathogens, including SARS-CoV-2, by employing this innovative strategy.

**Keywords:** Bioinformatics, COVID-19, Pathogen, Reverse vaccinology, SARS-CoV-2, Vaccine design.

## INTRODUCTION

Vaccines are one of the most successful and cost-effective prophylactic measures for improving the quality of health and saving lives from a wide range of infectious diseases worldwide [1, 2]. Eradication of smallpox and significant reduction of global polio cases are outstanding examples of successful vaccination programs where vaccines have significantly reduced mortality and the global burden of infectious diseases. Vaccines are weakened or attenuated from microorganisms or components, which, when introduced into an individual, stimulates the body's immune response and protects against an infectious disease

* **Corresponding author Arindam Mitra:** Department of Microbiology, School of Life Science and Biotechnology, Adamas University, Kolkata, India; Tel: +917305956643; E-mail: arindam.mitra@adamasuniversity.ac.in

**Parvesh Singh, Vipan Kumar & Rajshekhar Karpoormath (Eds.)**

caused by the pathogen or similar pathogens. Vaccinology focuses on vaccine development and the effect of vaccines on public health [3]. The classical steps of vaccine development include isolation, culture, and the weakening of a pathogen. Inoculation of a weakened or killed pathogen or a microbe component stimulates a protective immune response in the host. Purified components, such as capsules, recombinant proteins, or weakened toxins also confer protective immunity. Louis Pasteur designed this vaccinology approach of isolation, inactivation, and injection of the agent responsible for the disease. By reducing the pathogen's virulence or inhibiting the replication of a pathogen, the pathogen would be safer for hosts without compromising the immunogenicity of the pathogen. Targeting microbial components, such as capsules, toxins, and surface proteins, reduces the virulence of a given pathogen. This kind of vaccine strategy depends on the body's immune response to combat infectious diseases. It was successful against many infectious diseases such as smallpox, polio, mumps, measles, and rubella. Convalescent plasma therapy (CBT), also known as serum therapy or passive immune therapy, is another proven age-old therapeutic strategy. It depends on protective antibody responses from blood (sera and lymphocytes) from convalescent patients [4]. CBT treatment was successful against diphtheria, tetanus, pneumonia, anthrax, plague, tularemia, among many others [5]. In addition, this therapeutic strategy is employed against many emerging viral diseases, such as Ebola, SARS-CoV, and more recently against SARS-CoV-2 [6, 7]. Fig. (**1**) highlights classical approaches for vaccine development and convalescent plasma therapy against infectious diseases.

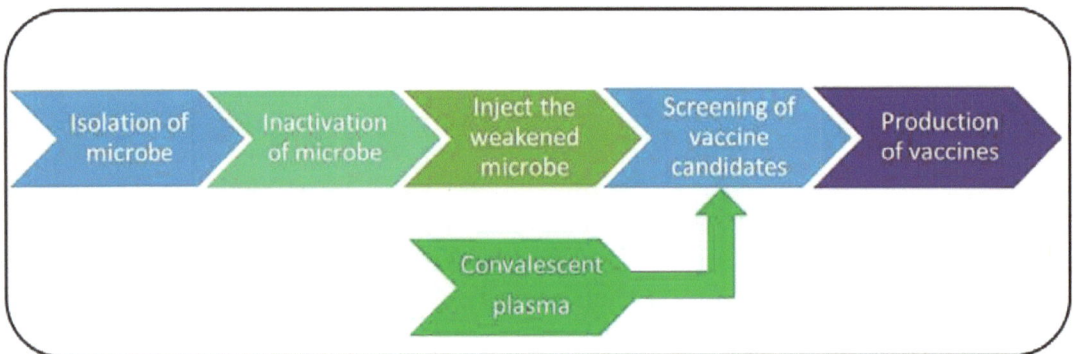

**Fig. (1).** Classical approaches for the development of vaccines and therapeutics.

However, there are certain limitations in the traditional approach for developing vaccines. Many infectious diseases such as tuberculosis, HIV, malaria, and others do not have an effective vaccine yet. In many cases, the development of a vaccine by the classical method is not feasible due to the lack of proper media for growing a given pathogen. It is difficult or not possible to express a given target antigen, as in meningitis and AIDS. The classical method is also not helpful in developing vaccines based on antigens that elicit strong autoimmune reactions or strains that are highly variable or where the mechanisms of pathogenesis are not well understood. Sometimes, the most expressed proteins may not be ideal vaccine candidates, or the antigens expressed *in vitro* are different from those expressed *in vivo*. Besides, the traditional method of developing vaccines can be time-consuming, and not all antigens can be made pure in adequate amounts for vaccine testing. Conventional vaccine development would not be effective against pathogens that do not induce immunity post-infection. The approach would not apply in cases of chronic diseases including AIDS, tuberculosis, gastritis and hepatitis [8].

## Reverse Vaccinology

The sequencing of the first microbe, *Haemophilus influenzae,* in 1995 opened up new possibilities for vaccine design [9]. With the availability of whole-genome sequence of many pathogens at an incredible speed using next-generation sequencing platforms, it is now possible to identify all potential protein antigens *in silico* that may be antigenic or immunogenic without actually culturing the pathogen. Using specific criteria of predictive algorithms and combining tools of bioinformatics and biotechnology, it is also possible to screen the exhaustive list of all potential antigens down to few candidate antigens that can eventually move to safety and immunogenicity testing. In many cases, secreted or extracellular antigens are more likely to be exposed to antibodies than intracellular protein antigens and are likely to be potential vaccine candidates.

Reverse Vaccinology (RV), a term coined by Rino Rappuoli, uses genomics and bioinformatics tools to develop vaccine candidates [10]. This approach enables the identification of all potential protective antigens from sequenced genomes. It facilitates the development of a safe and effective vaccine against any infectious disease that requires a protein antigen to stimulate an immune response [11 - 19]. Choice of algorithms, appropriate criteria for proper selection of antigens, and critical evaluation of the information often determine the success of the RV strategies. Genome-based approaches facilitate identifying novel antigens or unique virulence factors in pathogens, thereby enabling a better understanding of pathogenesis and developing better vaccines. RV-based vaccines are typically targeted based on specific purified components or subunit vaccines and not based on whole microbes. As a result, such vaccines do not elicit virulence or side effects, or adverse immune reactions from other microbial components. The conformations of epitopes designed by RV fold correctly due to the natural form of protein, and such epitopes can neutralize pathogens better than linear epitopes. RV approaches have reduced dependence on animal testing and clinical trials and are considered an economical approach to developing vaccines [20 - 22]. Fig. (**2**) outlines steps in reverse vaccinology.

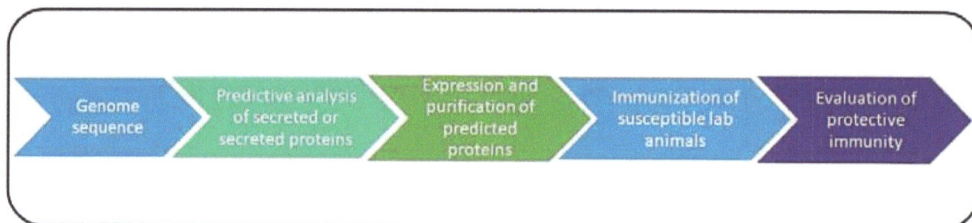

**Fig. (2).**  Reverse vaccinology steps for vaccine design.

## Vaccines Developed by Using Reverse Vaccinology

Reverse vaccinology successfully created a vaccine against *Neisseria meningitidis* serogroup B (Men B), causative agent of bacterial meningitis and sepsis, a lethal disease in children. It was extremely challenging to develop a vaccine against MenB because of the following reasons: the capsular polysaccharide of the pathogen was identical to human self-antigen, and the outer surface protein antigens were variable. However, with the availability of the genome sequence information, potential candidate antigens were screened based on the sequence information of *Neisseria* to develop vaccine candidates [23]. Based on predictive algorithms and a filtering approach using bioinformatics programs such as PSORTB, ProDorm, and Blocks database, 570 candidate membrane proteins or outer surface-exposed proteins have been identified. Out of those 570 candidates, recombinant DNA techniques could eventually clone 350 putative extracellular or surface-expressed proteins in *Escherichia coli*. Enzyme-Linked Immunosorbent Assay (ELISA) and Fluorescent-Activated Cell Sorting (FACS) confirmed the surface expressions of those candidate proteins. Subsequently, three hundred and fifty putative candidate antigens were injected into mice to raise antibodies against those antigens.

The researchers then evaluated the serum from immunized mice for bactericidal activity and complement activation. Antigen candidates were further screened based on conservation in multiple MenB strains to ensure broad protection against those strains, narrowing down to seven-candidate proteins. Eventually, three of seven proteins were used in the approved vaccine, BEXSERO, developed by Novartis to prevent the invasive disease caused by *Neisseria meningitidis* serogroup B [24] . Neisseria Heparin Binding Antigen, factor H binding protein, Neisseria adhesin A, and the outer membrane vesicles expressing porin A and porin B made into the vaccine, BEXSERO. Even though the initial assumption was that the vaccine would take a short period, but in reality, it took more than a decade to develop this vaccine. Also, an experimental vaccine based only on recombinant antigens was not successful. Hence, the final human vaccine is a combination of DNA technology and conventional vaccine technology. Nevertheless, the vaccine reduced the mortality and morbidity associated with the disease in European Union, Canada, and Australia and established the field of reverse vaccinology [25].

With this success, reverse vaccinology approaches were employed to design vaccines for many pathogens. Often appropriate modifications were made to RV strategies to meet specific objectives. For example, a multi-genome RV approach identified protective antigens from Group B streptococcus (GBS) instead of a single genome [26]. A subtractive RV approach identified unique antigens present in pathogenic *E. coli* but not in commensal *E. coli* [27]. Reverse vaccinology also helped develop vaccines against Hepatitis B, which is now routinely used to immunize children worldwide [28]. Furthermore, this technology successfully developed vaccines against emerging antibiotic-resistant pathogens such as *Staphylococcus aureus* and *Streptococcus pneumoniae* [19, 26, 29 - 32]. Tools, such as identifying open reading frames, homology searches, screening for cellular localization of proteins that span from the inner membrane to outside, and identifying surface-associated features, are used to pinpoint protective antigens based on genome analysis *in silico*. Usually, the genes encoding selected antigens are amplified, expressed in a heterologous system, and purified to generate a high level of potential protective antigens. Subsequently, the purified recombinant proteins are injected into mice. Later, the sera from animals are analyzed post-vaccination to verify the predicted surface association of antigens, and the protective immune response of those antigens is also analyzed. Table **1** summarizes recent reverse vaccinology approaches for vaccine design to combat many bacterial and viral pathogens [17, 19, 33 - 48].

Table 1. Recent reverse vaccinology approaches targeted against some emerging pathogens.

| Pathogen | Disease caused by the pathogen | Study/ Source |
|---|---|---|
| *Acinetobacter baumannii* | Urinary tract infections, pneumonia, wound infections | [33] |
| *Campylobacter jejuni* | Campylobacterosis | [34] |
| Nipah virus | Zoonotic disease affecting both humans and animals | [35] |
| *Salmonella enterica* serovar Typhi | Typhoid | [36] |

*(Table 1)  cont.....*

| Pathogen | Disease caused by the pathogen | Study/ Source |
|---|---|---|
| *Neisseria meningitidis* serogroup B | Meningitis | [37] |
| Hepatitis virus | Hepatitis | [38] |
| Avian Influenza virus | Diseases of the birds and can be pass to humans | [39] |
| *Staphylococcus aureus* | Skin infections, bloodstream infections, osteomyelitis | [19] |
| *Corynebacterium pseudotuberculosis* | Infection in horses, cattle, and ships | [40] |
| Japanese encephalitis virus | Infections of the brain | [41] |
| *Mycoplasma pneumoniae* | Infections of the respiratory system | [42] |
| *Shigella flexneri* | Shigellosis | [43] |
| *Vibrio cholerae* | Cholera | [44] |
| *Burkholderia pseudomallei* | Infections in humans or animals | [45] |
| *Plasmodium falciparum* | Malaria | [46] |
| Respiratory syncytial virus | Respiratory illness | [17] |
| SARS-CoV-2 | Respiratory illness | [47, 48] |

## Reverse Vaccinology for Intracellular Pathogens

*Rickettsia* is an intracellular bacterium that infects animals and humans worldwide and cannot be grown *in vitro*. The use of RV and molecular docking studies have facilitated the identification of vaccine candidates and drug targets against *Rickettsia* [49]. Another RV strategy identifies five MHC class 1 consensus epitopes of ornithine decarboxylase from *Leishmania donovani* [50]. *In silico* approach was used to predict protective antigens against melioidosis caused by *Burkholderia pseudomallei* [45, 51, 52]. State-of-the-art RV approaches could be employed to design vaccines against various neglected tropical diseases in resource-limited regions. These strategies could address biological complexity and low developmental costs associated with vaccine manufacturing [53].

The sequence information of many viruses due to enhanced next-generation sequencing methods made it possible to apply reverse vaccinology strategies towards viral vaccine development. The traditional method of selecting protective antigens against viral diseases relies on the notion that such antigens are typically expressed on the surface or secreted. As a result, many viral vaccines are being developed based on envelope and core proteins. Such a conventional strategy would fail to identify or ignore antigens expressed at insignificant levels or may not be part of the viral particle. RV strategies screen for protective antigens in the entire genome and minimize the inherent bias of using only specific available antigens. RV approaches also create a possibility of developing viral vaccines that are efficacious and timely, particularly for viruses relevant to public health as applicable in the current scenario [54].

## Reverse Vaccinology Strategies to Design A Vaccine Against SARS-CoV-2

Designing speedy and timely vaccines against SARS-CoV-2 *via* Reverse Vaccinology approaches opens up another practical approach for vaccine development in the context of the current pandemic of COVID-19. The current pandemic of Coronavirus Disease 2019, COVID-19, caused by Severe Acute Respiratory Syndrome Coronavirus 2 (SARS-CoV-2), causes severe pneumonia-like symptoms and shows high sequence similarity with SARS-CoV, which caused an earlier outbreak in 2002-03 [55]. The coronavirus is an enveloped, single-stranded, positive-sense RNA virus that causes severe respiratory diseases in humans. SARS-CoV-2 is a part of a family of beta Coronavirus and belongs to Coronaviridae, with characteristic crown-like projections on its surface, and its genome is fully sequenced [56]. The virus usually infects respiratory tracts in the human and other animals. The virus is thought to have a zoonotic origin in animals such as bats and later transmitted from humans to humans with a high reproductive number between 2 and 3. As of March 19, 2021, the pandemic resulted in 122M cases and 2.69M mortality globally. Several vaccine trials are currently in progress and few vaccines are in use. Still, a safe and efficacious vaccine to contain the SARS-CoV-2 would be desirable and bring normalcy. In this regard, reverse vaccinology strategies can offer a timely novel vaccine for a pathogen that may be difficult to grow in the lab. RV strategies can quickly develop a subunit vaccine against an emerging pathogen in a pandemic such as the one caused by SARS-CoV-2.

The complete genome sequence information of SARS-COV-2 is accessible (https://virological.org/t/novel-2019-coronavirus-genome/319).

Moreover, sequences of several other strains of the novel Coronavirus from different parts of the world are also available [57 - 59]. Various studies on vaccine development against SARS-CoV-2 using predictive tools are currently under investigation. Prediction of B cell epitope within the Spike Protein and T cell epitope within nucleocapsid protein using bioinformatics and immunoinformatic-based approaches has uncovered potential vaccine candidates against SARS-CoV- 2 [60]. Utilizing mass spectrometric-based predictive binding for HLA alleles, another study reported $CD4^+$ and $CD8^+T$ cell-binding epitopes to HLA-1 and HLA-2 alleles across the entire SARS-CoV-2 [61]. A Q-UEL language identifies a synthetic vaccine epitope and a peptidomimetic agent as potential candidates [62]. Structure-based immunoinformatic analysis of the S protein predicted multiple linear and non-linear B cell epitopes and T-cell epitopes [63, 64]. Investigators have also computationally predicted a stable multiple epitope vaccine using the spike protein of SARS-CoV-2 [65, 66]. E protein as a potential vaccine candidate is predicted based on bioinformatics approaches and modeling studies [67, 68]. Using *in silico* approaches, investigators have also designed multiple epitope fusion vaccine candidates that could elicit both humoral and cell-mediated immune responses against the novel Coronavirus [48]. A multi-epitope mRNA-based vaccine targets the spike protein based on immunoinformatic analysis for B and T cell epitopes, filtering, and molecular docking studies [69].

## Bioinformatics Based Vaccine Predictive Tools

Several bioinformatics analysis tools are available in the public domain to predict potential vaccine candidates using reverse vaccinology approaches. These tools typically use filtering or machine learning algorithms to make predictions. Vaxign was the first RV-based user-friendly web platform to predict antigens based on subcellular location and conservation and predict binding to MHC Class I and II [70, 71]. Machine learning has been applied to Vaxign further to create Vaxign-ML to predict better bacterial protective protein antigens [72, 73]. VirGen platform is a comprehensive viral genome resource with the structured organization of the genomic data [74]. EpiMatrix platform identifies and predicts epitopes [75]. Another platform, VIOLIN, is a vaccine-related database that stores, analyses, and integrates data on vaccine research [76, 77]. Vaceed is a high throughput platform to explore vaccine candidates against eukaryotic pathogens *in silico* [78]. VacSol is yet another high throughput platform to determine vaccine candidates against bacterial pathogens [79]. Jenner Predict server predicts vaccine candidates based on host-pathogen interactions and filters out cytosolic proteins [80]. VaxiJen is the first server-based immunogen prediction tool that relies solely on the physicochemical properties of proteins and is not dependent on the sequence alignment of proteins [81, 82]. ReVac is an RV-based predictive computational tool for protein-based bacterial vaccine candidates [83]. NERVE or New Enhanced Reverse Vaccinology Environment filters out proteins that may cause autoimmune reactions in humans [84]. Table **2** summarizes representative tools or web-based software programs used in Reverse vaccinology.

**Table 2. Representative predictive programs used in Reverse Vaccinology.**

| Programs | Utility | PMID/URL |
|---|---|---|
| Vaxign | First RV tool to make predictions of protein antigens based on subcellular location, conservation, and binding to MHC epitopes | http://www.violinet.org/vaxign/ |
| Vaxign-ML | Machine learning applied to Vaxign to make better predictions of antigens | http://www.violinet.org/vaxign/vaxign-ml/ |
| Vacceed | Makes prediction of antigens against eukaryotic pathogens | https://github.com/sgoodswe/vacceed/releases |
| NERVE | First automated RV approach with an autoimmunity filter | http://www.bio.unipd.it/molbinfo |
| Jenner predict | Predicts vaccine candidates based on host-pathogen interaction with cut off for cytosolic proteins | http://117.211.115.67/vaccine/home.html |
| Virgen | Comprehensive resource for viral genome and analysis | http://bioinfo.ernet.in/virgen/virgen.html |
| Epimatrix | Platform to identify and predict epitopes | https://epivax.com/immunogenicity-assessment/ivax-web-based-vaccine-design |
| Epitopemap | Web-based application for whole proteome epitope prediction | http://enzyme.ucd.ie/epitopemap |

*(Table 2) cont.....*

| Programs | Utility | PMID/URL |
|---|---|---|
| VIOLIN | Database for storing and retrieving information on vaccine research | http://www.violinet.org/ |
| VacSol | Predicts vaccine candidates against bacterial pathogens | https://bio.tools/vacsol |
| ReVac | Predicts protein-based vaccine candidates | https://github.com/admelloGithub/ReVac-package |

## Challenges of Reverse Vaccinology

The whole-genome sequence data of a pathogen is a prerequisite to reverse vaccinology. RV strategies also require an antibody-dependent response to a pathogen. The filtering approach in the selection of candidate antigen proteins introduces biases. Often, filtering predicts many surface-associated proteins as potential vaccine candidates, which then needs to be characterized and evaluated in the lab. In contrast, potential subcellular proteins are usually not considered as vaccine candidates. RV strategy is helpful if the vaccine candidate is protein-based and would not be effective if the vaccine is carbohydrate or lipid-based. The subunit vaccine candidates generated by RV approaches would specifically target against a component or components of a pathogen and not towards the whole pathogen. This strategy would provide a moderate level of immune response and may not offer long-term immunity, and might require the addition of adjuvants to boost the protective immunity in subunit vaccines.

## A Paradigm Shift in Vaccinology - Reverse Vaccinology 2.0

Several advances in human immunology and structural biology have been a major driving force for novel vaccine development and helped usher into a new era of Reverse Vaccinology 2.0 [85, 86]. A majority of vaccines confer a protective immune response by stimulation of pathogen-specific antibodies by B cells. Hence mechanisms of identifying pathogen-specific antibodies could assist the development of modern vaccines. Cloning B cells and producing recombinant monoclonal antibodies and antigen-binding fragments, screening most potent antibodies have enabled correct assessment of protective immune response. Structural vaccinology can improve the biochemical aspects and immunogenicity of vaccine candidates. Structure-based antigen design is the new frontier in vaccinology, and with this innovation, it is now possible to deliver antigens that were previously impossible. X-ray crystallography and NMR spectroscopy have greatly improved protein structure resolution and helped elucidate the structure and epitopes of most available vaccines [87]. Newer computational programming and approaches based on structural biology and immunology have greatly facilitated the identification of novel protective antigens [88]. Such advances in tools and technology have led us to an era of reverse vaccinology 2.0. Fig. (**3**) summarizes reverse vaccinology 2.0 approaches.

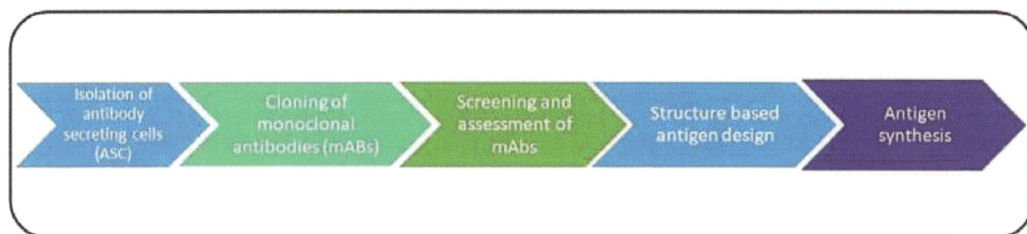

**Fig. (3).** Outline of Reverse Vaccinology 2.0.

## CONCLUSION

Reverse vaccinology offers novel ways to develop an efficacious vaccine in a relatively short period. It also enables high throughput expression of potential antigens and even circumvents pathogens' uncultivability problems. Many RV approaches are successful, and many vaccines are currently under development using such strategies. In the current pandemic, several researchers have used RV-based bioinformatics tools to predict potential antigens for developing vaccines to combat COVID-19. Newer strategies and technological developments supporting RV approaches include cloning B cells, high throughput expression of proteins, animal models, proteomics, antigen design, and structure-based design in vaccinology. Machine learning, deep learning, and molecular dynamics studies are also increasingly used to better construct protein antigens in the new era of Reverse Vaccinology 2.0. These technological innovations involving reverse vaccinology-based approaches are increasingly making a significant impact on designing vaccines to protect against diverse infectious diseases and emerging pathogens.

## CONSENT FOR PUBLICATION

Not applicable.

## CONFLICT OF INTEREST

The authors declare no conflict of interest, financial or otherwise.

## ACKNOWLEDGEMENTS

Declared none.

## REFERENCES

[1]     Vetter V, Denizer G, Friedland LR, Krishnan J, Shapiro M. Understanding modern-day vaccines: what you need to know. Ann Med 2018; 50(2): 110-20.
        [http://dx.doi.org/10.1080/07853890.2017.1407035] [PMID: 29172780]

[2]     Van der Zeijst BA. Vaccines and global stability: achievements and challenges. Expert Rev Vaccines 2008; 7(10): 1457-60.
        [http://dx.doi.org/10.1586/14760584.7.10.1457] [PMID: 19053201]

[3]     Pollard AJ, Bijker EM. A guide to vaccinology: from basic principles to new developments. Nat Rev Immunol 2021; 21(2): 83-100.
        [http://dx.doi.org/10.1038/s41577-020-00479-7] [PMID: 33353987]

[4]     Marano G, Vaglio S, Pupella S, *et al.* Convalescent plasma: new evidence for an old therapeutic tool? Blood Transfus 2016; 14(2): 152-7.
        [PMID: 26674811]

[5]     Manohar A, Ahuja J, Crane JK. Immunotherapy for infectious diseases: past, present, and future. Immunol Invest 2015; 44(8): 731-7.
        [http://dx.doi.org/10.3109/08820139.2015.1093914] [PMID: 26575462]

[6]     Walker LM, Burton DR. Passive immunotherapy of viral infections: 'super-antibodies' enter the fray. Nat Rev Immunol 2018; 18(5): 297-308.
        [http://dx.doi.org/10.1038/nri.2017.148] [PMID: 29379211]

[7]     Bloch EM, Shoham S, Casadevall A, *et al.* Deployment of convalescent plasma for the prevention and treatment of COVID-19. J Clin Invest 2020; 130(6): 2757-65.
        [http://dx.doi.org/10.1172/JCI138745] [PMID: 32254064]

[8]     Kennedy RB, Ovsyannikova IG, Palese P, Poland GA. Current challenges in vaccinology. Front Immunol 2020; 11: 1181.
        [http://dx.doi.org/10.3389/fimmu.2020.01181] [PMID: 32670279]

[9]     Fleischmann RD, Adams MD, White O, *et al.* Whole-genome random sequencing and assembly of Haemophilus influenzae Rd. Science 1995; 269(5223): 496-512.
        [http://dx.doi.org/10.1126/science.7542800] [PMID: 7542800]

[10]    Rappuoli R. Reverse vaccinology, a genome-based approach to vaccine development. Vaccine 2001; 19(17-19): 2688-91.
        [http://dx.doi.org/10.1016/S0264-410X(00)00554-5] [PMID: 11257410]

[11]    Hajialibeigi A, Amani J, Gargari SLM. Identification and evaluation of novel vaccine candidates against Shigella flexneri through reverse vaccinology approach. Appl Microbiol Biotechnol 2021; 105(3): 1159-73.
        [http://dx.doi.org/10.1007/s00253-020-11054-4] [PMID: 33452891]

[12]    Bibi S, Ullah I, Zhu B, *et al.* In silico analysis of epitope-based vaccine candidate against tuberculosis using reverse vaccinology. Sci Rep 2021; 11(1): 1249.
        [http://dx.doi.org/10.1038/s41598-020-80899-6] [PMID: 33441913]

[13]    Ashfaq UA, Saleem S, Masoud MS, *et al.* Rational design of multi epitope-based subunit vaccine by

exploring MERS-COV proteome: Reverse vaccinology and molecular docking approach. PLoS One 2021; 16(2): e0245072.
[http://dx.doi.org/10.1371/journal.pone.0245072] [PMID: 33534822]

[14]   Zilch TJ, Lee JJ, Bressan GC, *et al.* Evaluation of new leptospiral antigens for the diagnosis of equine leptospirosis: An approach using pan-genomic analysis, reverse vaccinology and antigenic selection. Equine Vet J 2020.
[http://dx.doi.org/10.1111/evj.13380] [PMID: 33135163]

[15]   Wang W, Liu J, Guo S, *et al.* Identification of *vibrio parahaemolyticus* and *vibrio* spp. specific outer membrane proteins by reverse vaccinology and surface proteome. Front Microbiol 2021; 11: 625315.
[http://dx.doi.org/10.3389/fmicb.2020.625315] [PMID: 33633699]

[16]   Ullah MA, Sarkar B, Islam SS. Exploiting the reverse vaccinology approach to design novel subunit vaccines against Ebola virus. Immunobiology 2020; 225(3): 151949.
[http://dx.doi.org/10.1016/j.imbio.2020.151949] [PMID: 32444135]

[17]   Tahir Ul Qamar M, Shokat Z, Muneer I, *et al.* Multiepitope-based subunit vaccine design and evaluation against respiratory syncytial virus using reverse vaccinology approach. Vaccines (Basel) 2020; 8(2): E288.
[http://dx.doi.org/10.3390/vaccines8020288] [PMID: 32521680]

[18]   Srivastava S, Sharma SK, Srivastava V, Kumar A. Proteomic exploration of *listeria monocytogenes* for the purpose of vaccine designing using a reverse vaccinology approach. Int J Pept Res Ther 2020; 1-21.
[PMID: 33144851]

[19]   Soltan MA, Magdy D, Solyman SM, Hanora A. Design of *staphylococcus aureus* new vaccine candidates with b and t cell epitope mapping, reverse vaccinology, and immunoinformatics. OMICS 2020; 24(4): 195-204.
[http://dx.doi.org/10.1089/omi.2019.0183] [PMID: 32286190]

[20]   Heinson AI, Woelk CH, Newell ML. The promise of reverse vaccinology. Int Health 2015; 7(2): 85-9.
[http://dx.doi.org/10.1093/inthealth/ihv002] [PMID: 25733557]

[21]   Del Tordello E, Rappuoli R, Delany I. Human vaccines. Academic Press 2017; pp. 65-86.
[http://dx.doi.org/10.1016/B978-0-12-802302-0.00002-9]

[22]   Donati C, Rappuoli R. Reverse vaccinology in the 21st century: improvements over the original design. Ann N Y Acad Sci 2013; 1285: 115-32.
[http://dx.doi.org/10.1111/nyas.12046] [PMID: 23527566]

[23]   Pizza M, Scarlato V, Masignani V, *et al.* Identification of vaccine candidates against serogroup B meningococcus by whole-genome sequencing. Science 2000; 287(5459): 1816-20.
[http://dx.doi.org/10.1126/science.287.5459.1816] [PMID: 10710308]

[24]   Serruto D, Bottomley MJ, Ram S, Giuliani MM, Rappuoli R. The new multicomponent vaccine against meningococcal serogroup B, 4CMenB: immunological, functional and structural characterization of the antigens. Vaccine 2012; 30 (Suppl. 2): B87-97.
[http://dx.doi.org/10.1016/j.vaccine.2012.01.033] [PMID: 22607904]

[25]   Watson PS, Turner DP. Clinical experience with the meningococcal B vaccine, Bexsero®: Prospects for reducing the burden of meningococcal serogroup B disease. Vaccine 2016; 34(7): 875-80.
[http://dx.doi.org/10.1016/j.vaccine.2015.11.057] [PMID: 26686570]

[26]   Maione D, Margarit I, Rinaudo CD, *et al.* Identification of a universal Group B streptococcus vaccine by multiple genome screen. Science 2005; 309(5731): 148-50.
[http://dx.doi.org/10.1126/science.1109869] [PMID: 15994562]

[27]   Rasko DA, Rosovitz MJ, Myers GS, *et al.* The pangenome structure of *Escherichia coli*: comparative genomic analysis of E. coli commensal and pathogenic isolates. J Bacteriol 2008; 190(20): 6881-93.
[http://dx.doi.org/10.1128/JB.00619-08] [PMID: 18676672]

[28]    Komatsu H. Hepatitis B virus: where do we stand and what is the next step for eradication? World J Gastroenterol 2014; 20(27): 8998-9016.
[PMID: 25083074]

[29]    Oprea M, Antohe F. Reverse-vaccinology strategy for designing T-cell epitope candidates for Staphylococcus aureus endocarditis vaccine. Biologicals 2013; 41(3): 148-53.
[http://dx.doi.org/10.1016/j.biologicals.2013.03.001] [PMID: 23582120]

[30]    Talukdar S, Zutshi S, Prashanth KS, Saikia KK, Kumar P. Identification of potential vaccine candidates against Streptococcus pneumoniae by reverse vaccinology approach. Appl Biochem Biotechnol 2014; 172(6): 3026-41.
[http://dx.doi.org/10.1007/s12010-014-0749-x] [PMID: 24482282]

[31]    Zhang Q, Lin K, Wang C, Xu Z, Yang L, Ma Q. Identification of Streptococcus mitis321A vaccine antigens based on reverse vaccinology. Mol Med Rep 2018; 17(6): 7477-86.
[http://dx.doi.org/10.3892/mmr.2018.8799] [PMID: 29620181]

[32]    Mamede LD, de Paula KG, de Oliveira B, *et al.* Reverse and structural vaccinology approach to design a highly immunogenic multi-epitope subunit vaccine against Streptococcus pneumoniae infection. Infect Genet Evol 2020; 85: 104473.
[http://dx.doi.org/10.1016/j.meegid.2020.104473] [PMID: 32712314]

[33]    Fereshteh S, Abdoli S, Shahcheraghi F, Ajdary S, Nazari M, Badmasti F. New putative vaccine candidates against Acinetobacter baumannii using the reverse vaccinology method. Microb Pathog 2020; 143: 104114.
[http://dx.doi.org/10.1016/j.micpath.2020.104114] [PMID: 32145321]

[34]    Gupta N, Kumar A. Designing an efficient multi-epitope vaccine against Campylobacter jejuni using immunoinformatics and reverse vaccinology approach. Microb Pathog 2020; 147: 104398.
[http://dx.doi.org/10.1016/j.micpath.2020.104398] [PMID: 32771659]

[35]    Krishnamoorthy PKP, Subasree S, Arthi U, Mobashir M, Gowda C, Revanasiddappa PD. T-cell epitope-based vaccine design for nipah virus by reverse vaccinology approach. Comb Chem High Throughput Screen 2020; 23(8): 788-96.
[http://dx.doi.org/10.2174/1386207323666200427114343] [PMID: 32338213]

[36]    Esmailnia E, Amani J, Gargari SLM. Identification of novel vaccine candidate against *Salmonella enterica* serovar Typhi by reverse vaccinology method and evaluation of its immunization. Genomics 2020; 112(5): 3374-81.
[http://dx.doi.org/10.1016/j.ygeno.2020.06.022] [PMID: 32565239]

[37]    Masignani V, Pizza M, Moxon ER. The development of a vaccine against meningococcus b using reverse vaccinology. Front Immunol 2019; 10: 751.
[http://dx.doi.org/10.3389/fimmu.2019.00751] [PMID: 31040844]

[38]    Chaudhuri D, Datta J, Majumder S, Giri K. In silico designing of peptide based vaccine for Hepatitis viruses using reverse vaccinology approach. Infect Genet Evol 2020; 84: 104388.
[http://dx.doi.org/10.1016/j.meegid.2020.104388] [PMID: 32485330]

[39]    Hasan M, Ghosh PP, Azim KF, *et al.* Reverse vaccinology approach to design a novel multi-epitope subunit vaccine against avian influenza A (H7N9) virus. Microb Pathog 2019; 130: 19-37.
[http://dx.doi.org/10.1016/j.micpath.2019.02.023] [PMID: 30822457]

[40]    Araújo CL, Alves J, Nogueira W, *et al.* Prediction of new vaccine targets in the core genome of Corynebacterium pseudotuberculosis through omics approaches and reverse vaccinology. Gene 2019; 702: 36-45.
[http://dx.doi.org/10.1016/j.gene.2019.03.049] [PMID: 30928361]

[41]    Chakraborty S, Barman A, Deb B. Japanese encephalitis virus: A multi-epitope loaded peptide vaccine formulation using reverse vaccinology approach. Infect Genet Evol 2020; 78: 104106.
[http://dx.doi.org/10.1016/j.meegid.2019.104106] [PMID: 31706079]

[42]    Vilela Rodrigues TC, Jaiswal AK, de Sarom A, *et al.* Reverse vaccinology and subtractive genomics reveal new therapeutic targets against *Mycoplasma pneumoniae*: a causative agent of pneumonia. R Soc Open Sci 2019; 6(7): 190907.
[http://dx.doi.org/10.1098/rsos.190907] [PMID: 31417766]

[43]    Leow CY, Kazi A, Hisyam Ismail CMK, *et al.* Reverse vaccinology approach for the identification and characterization of outer membrane proteins of *Shigella flexneri* as potential cellular- and antibody-dependent vaccine candidates. Clin Exp Vaccine Res 2020; 9(1): 15-25.
[http://dx.doi.org/10.7774/cevr.2020.9.1.15] [PMID: 32095437]

[44]    Rashid MI, Rehman S, Ali A, Andleeb S. Fishing for vaccines against *Vibrio cholerae* using *in silico* pan-proteomic reverse vaccinology approach. PeerJ 2019; 7: e6223.
[http://dx.doi.org/10.7717/peerj.6223] [PMID: 31249730]

[45]    Hizbullah , Nazir Z, Afridi SG, Shah M, Shams S, Khan A. Reverse vaccinology and subtractive genomics-based putative vaccine targets identification for Burkholderia pseudomallei Bp1651. Microb Pathog 2018; 125: 219-29.
[http://dx.doi.org/10.1016/j.micpath.2018.09.033] [PMID: 30243554]

[46]    Pritam M, Singh G, Swaroop S, Singh AK, Singh SP. Exploitation of reverse vaccinology and immunoinformatics as promising platform for genome-wide screening of new effective vaccine candidates against Plasmodium falciparum. BMC Bioinformatics 2019; 19 (Suppl. 13): 468.
[http://dx.doi.org/10.1186/s12859-018-2482-x] [PMID: 30717656]

[47]    Ong E, Wong MU, Huffman A, He Y. COVID-19 Coronavirus Vaccine Design Using Reverse Vaccinology and Machine Learning. Front Immunol 2020; 11: 1581.
[http://dx.doi.org/10.3389/fimmu.2020.01581] [PMID: 32719684]

[48]    Enayatkhani M, Hasaniazad M, Faezi S, *et al.* Reverse vaccinology approach to design a novel multi-epitope vaccine candidate against COVID-19: an in silico study. J Biomol Struct Dyn 2020; 1-16.
[http://dx.doi.org/10.1080/07391102.2020.1857843] [PMID: 32295479]

[49]    Felice AG, Alves LG, Freitas ASF, *et al.* Pan-genomic analyses of 47 complete genomes of the *Rickettsia* genus and prediction of new vaccine targets and virulence factors of the species. J Biomol Struct Dyn 2021; 1-15.
[PMID: 33719856]

[50]    Pandey RK, Dikhit MR, Lokhande KB, Pandey K, Das P, Bimal S. An immunoprophylactic evaluation of *Ld*-ODC derived HLA-A0201 restricted peptides against visceral leishmaniasis. J Biomol Struct Dyn 2021; 1-11.
[http://dx.doi.org/10.1080/07391102.2021.1876773] [PMID: 33602055]

[51]    Capelli R, Peri C, Villa R, *et al.* BPSL1626: reverse and structural vaccinology reveal a novel candidate for vaccine design against *Burkholderia pseudomallei*. Antibodies (Basel) 2018; 7(3): E26.
[http://dx.doi.org/10.3390/antib7030026] [PMID: 31544878]

[52]    Muruato LA, Tapia D, Hatcher CL, *et al.* Use of Reverse Vaccinology in the Design and Construction of Nanoglycoconjugate Vaccines against Burkholderia pseudomallei. Clin Vaccine Immunol 2017; 24(11): e00206-17.
[http://dx.doi.org/10.1128/CVI.00206-17] [PMID: 28903988]

[53]    Robleda-Castillo R, Ros-Lucas A, Martinez-Peinado N, Alonso-Padilla J. An overview of current uses and future opportunities for computer-assisted design of vaccines for neglected tropical diseases. Adv Appl Bioinform Chem 2021; 14: 25-47.
[http://dx.doi.org/10.2147/AABC.S258759] [PMID: 33623396]

[54]    Bruno L, Cortese M, Rappuoli R, Merola M. Lessons from Reverse Vaccinology for viral vaccine design. Curr Opin Virol 2015; 11: 89-97.
[http://dx.doi.org/10.1016/j.coviro.2015.03.001] [PMID: 25829256]

[55]    Petrosillo N, Viceconte G, Ergonul O, Ippolito G, Petersen E. COVID-19, SARS and MERS: are they

closely related? Clin Microbiol Infect 2020; 26(6): 729-34.
[http://dx.doi.org/10.1016/j.cmi.2020.03.026] [PMID: 32234451]

[56] Wu F, Zhao S, Yu B, *et al.* A new coronavirus associated with human respiratory disease in China. Nature 2020; 579(7798): 265-9.
[http://dx.doi.org/10.1038/s41586-020-2008-3] [PMID: 32015508]

[57] Sah R, Rodriguez-Morales AJ, Jha R, *et al.* Complete Genome Sequence of a 2019 Novel Coronavirus (SARS-CoV-2) Strain Isolated in Nepal. Microbiol Resour Announc 2020; 9(11): e00169-20.
[http://dx.doi.org/10.1128/MRA.00169-20] [PMID: 32165386]

[58] Padilla-Rojas C, Lope-Pari P, Vega-Chozo K, *et al.* Near-complete genome sequence of a 2019 novel coronavirus (SARS-CoV-2) strain causing a COVID-19 case in Peru. Microbiol Resour Announc 2020; 9(19): e00303-20.
[http://dx.doi.org/10.1128/MRA.00303-20] [PMID: 32381617]

[59] Lemriss S, Souiri A, Amar N, *et al.* Complete genome sequence of a 2019 novel coronavirus (sars-cov-2) strain causing a covid-19 case in Morocco. Microbiol Resour Announc 2020; 9(27): e00633-20.
[http://dx.doi.org/10.1128/MRA.00633-20] [PMID: 32616647]

[60] Chen HZ, Tang LL, Yu XL, Zhou J, Chang YF, Wu X. Bioinformatics analysis of epitope-based vaccine design against the novel SARS-CoV-2. Infect Dis Poverty 2020; 9(1): 88.
[http://dx.doi.org/10.1186/s40249-020-00713-3] [PMID: 32741372]

[61] Poran A, Harjanto D, Malloy M, *et al.* Sequence-based prediction of SARS-CoV-2 vaccine targets using a mass spectrometry-based bioinformatics predictor identifies immunogenic T cell epitopes. Genome Med 2020; 12(1): 70.
[http://dx.doi.org/10.1186/s13073-020-00767-w] [PMID: 32791978]

[62] Robson B. Computers and viral diseases. Preliminary bioinformatics studies on the design of a synthetic vaccine and a preventative peptidomimetic antagonist against the SARS-CoV-2 (2019-nCoV, COVID-19) coronavirus. Comput Biol Med 2020; 119: 103670.
[http://dx.doi.org/10.1016/j.compbiomed.2020.103670] [PMID: 32209231]

[63] Wang D, Mai J, Zhou W, *et al.* Immunoinformatic analysis of t- and b-cell epitopes for sars-cov-2 vaccine design. Vaccines (Basel) 2020; 8(3): E355.
[http://dx.doi.org/10.3390/vaccines8030355] [PMID: 32635180]

[64] Rahman N, Ali F, Basharat Z, *et al.* Vaccine design from the ensemble of surface glycoprotein epitopes of SARS-CoV-2: An immunoinformatics approach. Vaccines (Basel) 2020; 8(3): E423.
[http://dx.doi.org/10.3390/vaccines8030423] [PMID: 32731461]

[65] Kar T, Narsaria U, Basak S, *et al.* A candidate multi-epitope vaccine against SARS-CoV-2. Sci Rep 2020; 10(1): 10895.
[http://dx.doi.org/10.1038/s41598-020-67749-1] [PMID: 32616763]

[66] Lizbeth RG, Jazmín GM, José CB, Marlet MA. Immunoinformatics study to search epitopes of spike glycoprotein from SARS-CoV-2 as potential vaccine. J Biomol Struct Dyn 2020; 1-15.
[http://dx.doi.org/10.1080/07391102.2020.1780944] [PMID: 32583729]

[67] Sarkar M, Saha S. Structural insight into the role of novel SARS-CoV-2 E protein: A potential target for vaccine development and other therapeutic strategies. PLoS One 2020; 15(8): e0237300.
[http://dx.doi.org/10.1371/journal.pone.0237300] [PMID: 32785274]

[68] Ghafouri F, Cohan RA, Noorbakhsh F, Samimi H, Haghpanah V. An *in-silico* approach to develop of a multi-epitope vaccine candidate against SARS-CoV-2 envelope (E) protein. Res Sq 2020.

[69] Ahammad I, Lira SS. Designing a novel mRNA vaccine against SARS-CoV-2: An immunoinformatics approach. Int J Biol Macromol 2020; 162: 820-37.
[http://dx.doi.org/10.1016/j.ijbiomac.2020.06.213] [PMID: 32599237]

[70] Xiang Z, He Y. Genome-wide prediction of vaccine targets for human herpes simplex viruses using Vaxign reverse vaccinology. BMC Bioinformatics 2013; 14 (Suppl. 4): S2.

[http://dx.doi.org/10.1186/1471-2105-14-S4-S2] [PMID: 23514126]

[71]   He Y, Xiang Z, Mobley HL. Vaxign: the first web-based vaccine design program for reverse vaccinology and applications for vaccine development. J Biomed Biotechnol 2010; 2010: 297505.
[http://dx.doi.org/10.1155/2010/297505] [PMID: 20671958]

[72]   Ong E, Wang H, Wong MU, Seetharaman M, Valdez N, He Y. Vaxign-ML: supervised machine learning reverse vaccinology model for improved prediction of bacterial protective antigens. Bioinformatics 2020; 36(10): 3185-91.
[http://dx.doi.org/10.1093/bioinformatics/btaa119] [PMID: 32096826]

[73]   Bowman BN, McAdam PR, Vivona S, *et al.* Improving reverse vaccinology with a machine learning approach. Vaccine 2011; 29(45): 8156-64.
[http://dx.doi.org/10.1016/j.vaccine.2011.07.142] [PMID: 21864619]

[74]   Kulkarni-Kale U, Bhosle S, Manjari GS, Kolaskar AS. VirGen: a comprehensive viral genome resource. Nucleic Acids Res 2004; 32(Database issue): D289-92.
[http://dx.doi.org/10.1093/nar/gkh098] [PMID: 14681415]

[75]   De Groot AS, Jesdale BM, Szu E, Schafer JR, Chicz RM, Deocampo G. An interactive Web site providing major histocompatibility ligand predictions: application to HIV research. AIDS Res Hum Retroviruses 1997; 13(7): 529-31.
[http://dx.doi.org/10.1089/aid.1997.13.529] [PMID: 9135870]

[76]   He Y, Racz R, Sayers S, *et al.* Updates on the web-based VIOLIN vaccine database and analysis system. Nucleic Acids Res 2014; 42(Database issue): D1124-32.
[http://dx.doi.org/10.1093/nar/gkt1133] [PMID: 24259431]

[77]   Xiang Z, Todd T, Ku KP, *et al.* VIOLIN: vaccine investigation and online information network. Nucleic Acids Res 2008; 36(Database issue): D923-8.
[PMID: 18025042]

[78]   Goodswen SJ, Kennedy PJ, Ellis JT. Vacceed: a high-throughput *in silico* vaccine candidate discovery pipeline for eukaryotic pathogens based on reverse vaccinology. Bioinformatics 2014; 30(16): 2381-3.
[http://dx.doi.org/10.1093/bioinformatics/btu300] [PMID: 24790156]

[79]   Rizwan M, Naz A, Ahmad J, *et al.* VacSol: a high throughput in silico pipeline to predict potential therapeutic targets in prokaryotic pathogens using subtractive reverse vaccinology. BMC Bioinformatics 2017; 18(1): 106.
[http://dx.doi.org/10.1186/s12859-017-1540-0] [PMID: 28193166]

[80]   Jaiswal V, Chanumolu SK, Gupta A, Chauhan RS, Rout C. Jenner-predict server: prediction of protein vaccine candidates (PVCs) in bacteria based on host-pathogen interactions. BMC Bioinformatics 2013; 14: 211.
[http://dx.doi.org/10.1186/1471-2105-14-211] [PMID: 23815072]

[81]   Zaharieva N, Dimitrov I, Flower DR, Doytchinova I. Vaxijen dataset of bacterial immunogens: An update. Curr Computeraided Drug Des 2019; 15(5): 398-400.
[http://dx.doi.org/10.2174/1573409915666190318121838] [PMID: 30887928]

[82]   Doytchinova IA, Flower DR. VaxiJen: a server for prediction of protective antigens, tumour antigens and subunit vaccines. BMC Bioinformatics 2007; 8: 4.
[http://dx.doi.org/10.1186/1471-2105-8-4] [PMID: 17207271]

[83]   D'Mello A, Ahearn CP, Murphy TF, Tettelin H. ReVac: a reverse vaccinology computational pipeline for prioritization of prokaryotic protein vaccine candidates. BMC Genomics 2019; 20(1): 981.
[http://dx.doi.org/10.1186/s12864-019-6195-y] [PMID: 31842745]

[84]   Vivona S, Bernante F, Filippini F. NERVE: new enhanced reverse vaccinology environment. BMC Biotechnol 2006; 6: 35.
[http://dx.doi.org/10.1186/1472-6750-6-35] [PMID: 16848907]

[85]   Burton DR. What are the most powerful immunogen design vaccine strategies? reverse vaccinology

2.0 shows great promise. Cold Spring Harb Perspect Biol 2017; 9(11): a030262.
[http://dx.doi.org/10.1101/cshperspect.a030262] [PMID: 28159875]

[86]    Bidmos FA, Siris S, Gladstone CA, Langford PR. Bacterial vaccine antigen discovery in the reverse vaccinology 2.0 era: Progress and challenges. Front Immunol 2018; 9: 2315.
[http://dx.doi.org/10.3389/fimmu.2018.02315] [PMID: 30349542]

[87]    Dormitzer PR, Grandi G, Rappuoli R. Structural vaccinology starts to deliver. Nat Rev Microbiol 2012; 10(12): 807-13.
[http://dx.doi.org/10.1038/nrmicro2893] [PMID: 23154260]

[88]    Rappuoli R, Bottomley MJ, D'Oro U, Finco O, De Gregorio E. Reverse vaccinology 2.0: Human immunology instructs vaccine antigen design. J Exp Med 2016; 213(4): 469-81.
[http://dx.doi.org/10.1084/jem.20151960] [PMID: 27022144]

# CHAPTER 2

# Leptospirosis - A Complete Review

**N. Ramalakshmi[1,*], S. Arunkumar[2] and A. Puratchikody[3]**

[1] *C.L Baid Metha College of Pharmacy, Chennai, India*

[2] *School of Pharmacy, Satyabama Institute of Science and Technology, Chennai, India*

[3] *University College of Engineering, Bharathidasan Institute of Technology Campus, Anna University, Tiruchirappalli, India*

**Abstract:** Leptospirosis is a rare but neglected bacterial infection that affects people and animals. It is caused by bacteria of the genus *Leptospira*. The disease was reported as early as 1886 by Adolf Weil. Leptospirosis may cause kidney damage, meningitis, liver failure, respiratory distress, and even death when it is not treated. Occupations at risk include surfers, slaughterhouse workers, farmers, sewer workers and, people working on derelict buildings. Amjad Islam *et al.* had reported that among Asian countries, its highest prevalence is found in India. In 2015, Federico Costa *et al.* estimated that leptospirosis causes 1.03 million cases worldwide each year. The pooled mortality rate is 25%. WHO has estimated that 0.1 to 1 per 100 000 people living in temperate climates are affected each year, with the number increasing to 10 or more per 100 000 people living in tropical climates. It is reported in all continents except Antarctica. Lesser availability of treatment resources is detrimental, and unfortunately, it is commonly reported in lower-middle-income group countries.

The current treatment modalities for milder cases of leptospirosis rely on antibiotic administration viz penicillin, ampicillin, cefmetazole, oxalactam, ceftizoxime, and cefotaxime.

Whereas, in severe cases, intravenous penicillin G has long been the drug of choice; the patients treated with penicillin for the management of this disease are to be monitored throughout the treatment to prevent the severe threat of potential Jarisch-Herxheimer reactions. In particular, this immune-mediated hypersensitivity reaction may occur within 4-5 h after administration of penicillins. Various kinds of human leptospirosis vaccines have been developed, including inactivated whole-cell, outer-envelope, and recombinant vaccines. Of these, only a multivalent inactivated leptospirosis vaccine (killed vaccine) is available in China, Japan, and Vietnam. However, human vaccines for leptospirosis are serovar-specific and require yearly boosters. So there is a need for the development of novel compounds which have leptospirocidal activity. Notably, drugs for treating leptospirosis are minimum; the present research for the development of novel lead compounds for this pathogen is very limited.

**\* Correspondence author N. Ramalakshmi:** C.L Baid Metha College of Pharmacy, Chennai, India; Tel: +91 9840975248; E-mail: ramalakshmi.arunkumar@gmail.com

**Parvesh Singh, Vipan Kumar & Rajshekhar Karpoormath (Eds.)**

This review aims to summarize the most recent literature on synthetic lead molecules, natural products for its treatment, drug targets, *etc.*, and provide recommendations to researchers who may encounter difficulties in finding details on the subject.

**Keywords:** Drug targets, Leptospirosis, Natural products, Synthetic analogs.

## HISTORY OF LEPTOSPIROSIS

Leptospirosis is caused by the pathogenic bacteria of the genus Leptospira. This zoonotic disease is prevalent in every continent, except in the Polar regions. The tropical climate has highly favorable ecological conditions for transmission of leptospirosis than temperate climate. Even if leptospirosis is primarily considered a tropical disease, it is ubiquitously present in temperate climates due to changes in environmental conditions, and the migration of humans. As a consequence of ever-increasing awareness and high case incidence, this disease has been scheduled as an emerging global public health disease [1]. It is primarily transmitted through water, food, soil, and mud contaminated with the urine of infected animals to the human. When bacteria enter through skin abrasions and mucous membranes of the mouth, eyes, and nose, humans can acquire leptospirosis.

Leptospirosis was recognized as an occupational hazard of rice harvesters in ancient China. In Japan, leptospirosis was termed as *akiyami*, or autumn fever. Larrey, in 1812, identified leptospirosis as fièvrejaune among Napoleon's troops at the siege of Cairo in Egypt. Initially, the endemic disease was supposed to be related to the plague but not as contagious. About 100 years ago, workers in Japan and Europe contemporarily isolated Leptospira and identified it as a causative agent for the classical syndrome, the Weil's disease. The nineteenth-century brought rational insights into the cause for the outbreak of icteric fever, which was also called by other names like Griesinger's bilious typhoid, bilious or hepatic fever, hepatic typhoid, icteric typhoid, catarrhal icterus, and febrile icterus. Later on, the icteric infection was known as Weil's disease, and it occurs when humans are exposed to direct contact with water, marshy land, wet soil, or mud. In 1879, spirochete species of the Borrelia genus were the cause of relapsing fever of leptospirosis. Spirochaetes, later to be identified as leptospires, were discovered by Japanese investigators in field mice and rats in 1915 [2]. Leptospires were isolated from leptospirosis patients that occurred as mixed infections with yellow fever [3, 4]. In the beginning, it was thought that dengue, sandfly fever, and leptospirosis were caused by the same organism. But later, it was confirmed that dengue and sandfly fever were caused by flavivirus and phlebovirus, respectively, and not by leptospirosis [5].

In Western Europe, *Leptospirainterrogans* serovars icterohaemorrhagiae was introduced in the 18th century by the westward extension of the range of *Rattusnorvegicus* from Eurasia [6]. There was a report published in the landmark Institute of Medicine entitled "Emerging Infections: Microbial Threats to Health in the United States"; herein, leptospirosis was used as an example of an infection that had in the past caused significant morbidity in military personnel deployed in tropical areas [7]. A new infectious disease was identified from cattle in Georgia in 1935. This infection was associated with icterus, bloody urine, and skin necrosis. The mortality rate ranged between 10 and 60 percent. In 1938, it was reported convalescent serum from such infected cattle agglutinated Leptospira grippotyphosa in high titer. It was found that the disease was transmitted by mice. Convalescent sera served as an effective means of treatment [8, 9].

Veterinarians, farmers, sewer workers are at high risk of contracting the disease. Recreational activities involving freshwater, foreign travel, or a combination of both spike the chances of being infected with leptospirosis infection [10]. During World War I, outbreaks were confirmed in French, German, and British troops [11]. This is due to favorable conditions conferred by trench warfare which include water and rat manifestation. "Fort Bragg Fever", a form of leptospirosis, led to hospitalization of 40 soldiers at Ft. Bragg in North Carolina in the summer of 1942 [12]. In 1961, US military troops were also infected with the pathogen. In 1987, Japanese troops were infected during a water-borne outbreak in Okinawa [13].

Recently, a surge has been witnessed in the number of leptospirosis cases partly due to incessant rain, environmental factors such as polluted water, poor waste management, *etc.* in Ernakulam district, Kerala India. Despite the availability of a drug with proven efficacy as prophylactic against leptospirosis, the refusal of people to take the drug, given at free of cost continues to baffle the district health department [14].

## EPIDEMIOLOGY

Epidemiological studies on this subject have been conducted worldwide with the purpose to understand the types of risk factors associated with this disease, and what action needs to be taken to prevent further spread out. However, no answers have been provided as to what causes this illness to a specific individual.

The higher incidence of leptospirosis is located in tropical countries like Latin America, India, Southeast Asia [15, 16]. The division of WHO known as Leptospirosis Burden Epidemiology Reference Group (LERG) conducted a systematic literature review that estimated global annual incidence of endemic and epidemic human leptospirosis, which resulted in varying from 5 to 14 cases per 100,000 [17]. Rodents, in particular rats, are the main reservoir for the circulation of leptospirosis in the environment. Leptospirosis is known to be endemic in India since the early 20th century. The primary source of leptospirosis is the excreta of animal, from whose renal tubules leptospires are excreted through the urine to the environment [18, 19]. The predominating risk factor for humans is their occupation. Direct contact with infected animals accounts for inspectors. The highest risk is associated with swine farming, slaughterhouse, and meat industry workers [20].

An epidemiological investigation was carried out in Barbados, a country in the Caribbean Sea. This survey revealed the seroprevalence of Leptospirosis in the various occupational groups to be 29.8% (highest in sanitation workers – 42.7%, followed by sugarcane workers – 39.4%) [21]. A high prevalence of leptospiral antibodies in humans was reported from Somalia in 1982 [22]. The sero prevalence of leptospirosis in jaundice patients was reported in Madras in1983 [23, 24]. In 1987, Seroprevalence was reported in Karachi [25], and in 1989, it was reported in Barbados school children [26]. In 1984 to 1985, leptospirosis in 19 humans was reported in Madras [27]. In 1993, it was reported in Diglipur of North Andamans [28]. In 1996, five patients in the Illinois Department of Public Health were notified with an unknown febrile illness after participation in a white-water rafting trip on flooded rivers in Costa Rica. An outbreak of leptospirosis was found amidst athletes and community workers after their involvement in triathlons was held in Springfield, Illinois [29]. A review of epidemiological studies will channelize interventions for health and environmental control in the area of the neglected disease.

## MORPHOLOGY

Leptospira are cork-shaped spirochaetes, and they differ from other spirochaetes by the presence of end hooks (Fig. 1). They are highly motile aerobic spirochetes. This spirochaete has 2 periplasmic flagella which are responsible for their mobility. They possess a double membrane structure which has a cytoplasmic membrane and a peptidoglycan cell wall. They contain lipopolysaccharide in their cell membrane [30].

They appear with common laboratory stains and are best visualized by darkfield microscopy, silver stain, or fluorescent microscopy [31]. Replication of leptospires in many animal hosts probably takes place at 37°C or higher, yet efficient laboratory propagation demands incubation at 29-30°C [32].

The genus Leptospira was historically classified into two species, Leptospira interrogans and *L. biflexa*, which comprise pathogenic and non-pathogenic strains, respectively.

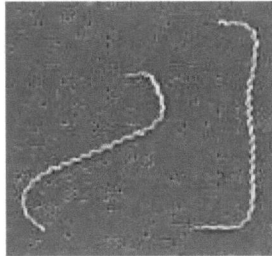

**Fig. (1).**  Morphology of Leptospira.

## CLINICAL FEATURES OF LEPTOSPIROSIS

The Centre for disease control and prevention, USA, stated that this disease may occur in two phases:

- During the first phase, the patients may possess indications such as fever, chills, headache, muscle aches, vomiting, or diarrhea, and after that, the patient may recover for a time but become sick yet again.
- The second phase is more rigorous. The patient may have kidney or liver failure, or meningitis.

This illness lasts for a few days to 3 weeks or longer. Without treatment, recovery may take several months.

The important characteristic of Weil disease is Hemorrhagic manifestation. The Leptospira toxins induce hemodynamic abnormalities in patients, secondary to hypovolemia. This fatal condition is caused by the loss of extracellular fluid and the direct effects of bacterial *toxins* that damage vascular endothelium and increase permeability. In human leptospirosis, the manifestation of hemorrhage is increasingly reported over the world. As a result of a defect in the primary hemostasis or an imbalance in secondary hemostasis, bleeding may occur in patients. This may be due to enhanced coagulation or activated fibrinolysis that causes depletion of coagulation proteins. Other indications include thrombocytopenia, the elevation of serum bilirubin, hematuria, and pulmonary hemorrhage [33]. The pathogenic leptospires invade the intercellular junctions of host hepatocytes and cause hepatocyte apoptosis [34].

## CURRENT TREATMENT

Outpatients with mild cases of Leptospirosis are treated with antibiotics, such as doxycycline or azithromycin. In pregnant women, it can be treated with either azithromycin or amoxicillin. In the case of hospitalised adults with severe disease, treatment with penicillin, doxycycline, ceftriaxone or cefotaxime is preferred. Whereas, for children who cannot tolerate the above agents, azithromycin is an acceptable alternative agent. Pregnant women with severe leptospirosis may be treated with penicillin, ceftriaxone, cefotaxime, and azithromycin. Doxycycline appears to be safer in pregnancy than tetracyclines. The duration of treatment in severe disease is usually seven days.

The patients treated with penicillin for the management of this disease are to be monitored throughout the treatment to prevent the severe threat of potential Jarisch-Herxheimer reactions. This immune-mediated hypersensitivity reaction may occur within 4-5 h after administration of penicillins.

A very few countries use vaccines for the treatment of leptospirosis. In United States of America, there are no commercially available vaccines. Various kinds of human leptospirosis vaccines have been developed including inactivated whole-cell, outer-envelope, and recombinant vaccines. Of these, only a multivalent inactivated leptospirosis vaccine (killed vaccine) is available in China, Japan, and Vietnam.


## DRUG TARGETS

Lipopolysaccharides and peptidoglycan biosynthesis are the two major pathogen-specific pathways. Eight enzymes of the lipopolysaccharide pathway (LpxB, LpxC, LpxD, KdsA, KdsB1, GmhA, KdtA, and RfaE2) and seven enzymes of the peptidoglycan biosynthesis pathway (MurA, MurC, MurD, MurE, MurF, MurG, and Ddl) were identified as a potential common drug target in the study carried out by U. Amineni *et al*. [33].

Reena Gupta *et al*. had reported 34 common drug targets.

Various drug targets for leptospirosis are as follows:

Drug target

1. PdXA involved in pyridoxal phosphate biosynthesis

2. Phosphoadenosinephosphosulphatereductase

3. NAD- dependent protein deacylase

4. 3-methyl-2-oxo butanoate hydroxyl methyl transferase

5. Homoserine O acetyl transferase

6. Acyl[acyl carrier protein] UDP N-acetyl glucosamine O-transferase

7. Lipid A disaccharide synthetase

8. 6,7-dimethyl-8-ribityl lumazine synthase

9. Tetra acyldisaccharide4'kianase

10. Thiamine phosphate kianase

11. Sulfate adenyltransferase

12. 3-deoxymanno-octo losonatecytidyltransferase

13. Aspartate alpha decarboxylase

14. UDP-N-acetylglucosamine-2 epimerase

15. Mannose-6-phosphate isomerase.

16. N-(5'-phosphoribosyl) anthranilateisomerase

17. Pantoate beta alanine ligase

18. Glutamate cysteine ligase

19. 3-deoxymanno-octo losonatic acid transferase

20. UDP-3-O-(3-hydroxymyrsitoyl) N-acetylglucosaminedeacetylase

21. UDP-3-O-(3-hydroxymyrsitoyl) N-acetylglucosamine acyl transferase

22. 4-hydroxy benzoate octaprenyltransferase

23. 3-polyprenyl-4-hydroxy benzoate decarboxylase

24. Phosphoheptoseisomerase

25. Pyridoxine-5' phosphate synthase

26. UDP-N-acetyl glucosamine diphosphorylase

27. NAD-dependendant-7-cyano-7-deazaguanine reductase

28. Cob(1) alamin adenosyl transferase

29. Dehypoxanthine futalosine cyclase

30. L-lysine2,3-aminomutase

31. Methylase of chemotaxis methyl accepting protein

32. Flagellar motar switch protein

33. MCP-methylation inhibitor.

34. Two -component system histidine kinase.

Also, they had explored two more important target enzymes in their study [34].

The cobA with an EC: 2.5.1.17 participated in the cobalamin biosynthesis pathway. Pathogenic strains of *Leptospira* can't grow in the absence of cobalamin that's why it is an essential component of the Ellinghausen-McCullough-Johns-n-Harris (EMJH) semi-synthetic selective medium. In contrast, gene thiL was found to be important in the conversion of thiamine monophosphate to thiamine pyrophosphate which is essential for the pathogen survival.

Outer membrane proteins (OMP) are important for the interaction of pathogen with host immune cells. KS Latha *et al* identified 21 OMPs in their research and they have reported that among the 21 proteins, 2 proteins with UniProt ID: Q75FL0 and Q72PD2 play a crucial role [35]

Peptide deformylase is an essential bacterial metalloproteinase enzyme. It plays an important role in removing the formal group from N-terminal methionine which is essential for the survival of bacteria [36]. Nally *et al* showed that LoA22, an outer lipoprotein important for virulence, LipL32, LipL41 are also very important for irulence [37].LipL32, LigA, LigB, LipL21 and LoA22 are lipoproteins which are thought to be adhesins, binding cells or different components of the extracellular matrix [6]. KDO (2-keto-3-deoxyma-no-octulosonic acid) is an eight-carbon acidic sugar found in the LPS of Gramnegative bacteria and it connects the Lipid A part to the O-antigen [38]. So this can be an important target in designing novel design of drugs for leptospirosis. UDP-3-O-acyl-N-acetylglucosamine deacetylase (LpxC) is a Zn-dependent protein that participates in the biosynthesis of lipid A. Lipid A anchors lipopolysaccharides into the membrane of Gram-negative bacteria. LpxC catalyzes the conversion of UDP-3-O-[(3R)-3- hydroxymyristoyl ]-N-acetyl glucosamine to UDP-3- O-[ (3R)-3-hydroxymy ristoy l]- N-glucosamine [39]. LRR protein LIC10831 was identified as a drug target for leptospirosis by Shepard *et al.*, [40]. Bacterial secretome plays an essential role as virulence factors pathogenicity, such as host-pathogen interactions, Preliminary MS analysis of secretomes found 29 proteins ranging from 8.7 to 95 kDa . They are classically sec-dependent type I and II SPase SE *i.e.*, hypothetical protein, outer membrane protein, lipoprotein, several enzymes (serine O-acetyltransferase, DNA helicase, dihydrolipoamide dehydrogenase, tRNA ligase, ATP-dependent Clp protease, ADP-heptose synthase, trypsin-like serine protease, glycerol--phosphate dehydrogenase, methyltransferase and lysine decarboxylase), and others proteins.

UDP N-acetyl glucosamine N-acetylmuramyl (pentapeptide) pyrophosphoryl-undecaprenol N-acetylglucosaminetransferase is an important protein in peptidoglycan synthesis. This could be an important drug target in leptospirosis [41]. OmpL1 is the first transmembrane OMP described from a pathogenic spirochete. OmpL1 was originally isolated in surface immunoprecipitation studies intended to identify proteins exposed on the leptospiral surface [42]. LipL32 protein of pathogenic leptospiral species is also reported as an important target for leptospirosis. NIC protein: LipL32 is the major leptospiral antigenic protein present in the outer membrane of the pathogen [43 - 45].

## CURRENTLY AVAILABLE DIAGNOSTIC TESTS

Serological diagnosis is used to diagnose most of the leptospiral cases. Antibodies for the pathogen are detected after 5 to 7 days. Genus specific and serogroup specific are the two methods of serological testing. After the isolation of the organism agglutination tests were described [46]. The microscopic agglutination test is the most important method to detect the pathogen. MAT test requires live cultures of all for use as antigens. Patient sera are reacted with this live antigen and incubated. After incubation the mixture is microscopically examined for agglutination under darkfield microscopy. The end point is the highest dilution of serum at which 50% agglutination occurs [47].

In another serological test the antibodies were detected using an IgM enzyme-linked immunosorbent assay (ELISA), an IgM-dipstick assay, and a hemagglutination assay IHA.

### IgM-Enzyme Linked Immunosorbent Assay

Test sera, cutoff calibrator, positive and negative control sera were diluted 1:100 in serum diluent, and 100 μL added to *Leptospira* antigen-coated microwells and incubated for 30 minutes at 37°C. After washing with phosphate-buffered saline containing 0.05% Tween 20, 100 µL of HRP conjugated anti-human IgM was added and incubated for another 30 minutes at 37°C. After further washing, 100 µL of tetramethylbenzidine substrate was added and incubated at room temperature for 10 minutes, after which the reaction was stopped with 100 µL of 1 M phosphoric acid. The absorbance of each well is read at a wavelength of 450 nm with a Bio-Tek ELX 808 plate reader (Bio-Tek Instruments, Winooski, VT). The results were expressed as Panbio units calculated by the ratio of sample absorbance to the mean cutoff absorbance multiplied by 10 [48].

## IgM-dipstick Assay

The assay is based on the binding of human Leptospira-specific **IgM** antibodies to the Leptospira antigen. Bound **IgM** antibodies are specifically detected with an anti-human **IgM** dye conjugate. The broadly reactive Leptospira antigen ensures the efficient detection of a wide spectrum of Leptospira infections [49]

## The Indirect Hemagglutination Assay (IHA)

This method uses a soluble antigen from serotype Patoc to sensitize sheep erythrocytes, which are then fixed with glutaraldehyde. The sensitized fixed erythrocytes may be stored for at least one year [50]

Other tests include radio immuno assay method [51], immune florescence [52], counter immune electrophoresis [53], and thin layer immune assay [54].

## Molecular Diagnosis

Dot blotting and in situ hybridization are the most important techniques for Leptospiral DNA identification [55]. However, PCR technique was found to be the most successful method for the detection of leptospires. Some PCR technique is based on specific gene targets like 16S or and 23 S rRNA genes while others are based on genomic libraries

## Molecular Typing

Because of the difficulties associated with serological identification of leptospiral isolates, there has been great interest in molecular methods for identification and subtyping. Methods employed have included digestion of chromosomal DNA by restriction endonucleases (REA), restriction fragment length polymorphism (RFLP), ribotyping, PFGE, and several PCR-based approaches [56].

## NATURAL PRODUCTS FOR THE TREATMENT OF LEPTOSPIROSIS

Since the therapies for curing Leptospira in modern medicine are very limited, potential alternatives from traditional medicine and their mechanisms of action are worth investigating. In recent years, there has been a global trend towards the use of natural phytochemicals such as herbs, fruits, and vegetables as antioxidant agents. India is a vast country having botanical and mineral wealth and also abundant flora and fauna. About 80% of Indian population depends on traditional system of medicines because of severe adverse reactions experienced by conventional medicines and other reasons.

Six plant-derived compounds from the leaves of an endemic plant *Glyptopetalum calocarpum* was evaluated for antileptospiral activity by Punnam chander *et al.* wo. Out of six compounds, two compounds namely namely lupenone and stigmasterol, showed anti-leptospiral activity and minimum inhibitory concentrations of the two compounds tested against pathogenic leptospiral strains belonging to 10 serovars were in the range of 100-200 µg/mL [57]. Other four compounds, namely α lupene, lupeol, β-amyrin and β-amyrin acetate, did not show any activity within the range of concentrations tested.

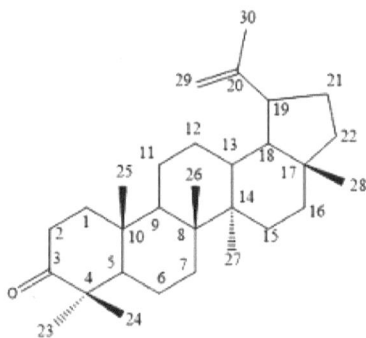

Lupenone

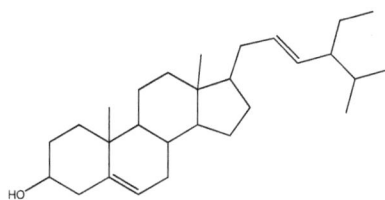

stigmasterol

The ethanolic extract of *Eclipta alba* L. showed anti leptospirocidal activity against various sero groups of *Leptospira interrogans*. *L. australis, L. autumnalis* and *L. grippotyphosa* are inhibited by both water and ethanol extract by tube dilution technique. The MIC level observed are 50 µg and 100 µg respectively [58]. Chandan *et al.*, selected DNA of *L. icterohaemorrhagiae* to study DNA cleavage and exposure of the DNA of *L. icterohaemorrhagiae* to *Eclipta alba* and *Phyllanthus amarus* plant extracts resulted in DNA cleavage. The fact that the organic solvent extracts exhibited greater anti*Leptospiral* activity and this is because the antimicrobial principles were either polar or non-polar and they were extracted only through the organic solvent medium [59]

Andrographis paniculata Nees (Acanthaceae) was evaluated by Arulmozhi and Natarajasreenivasan for 1 antileptospiral activity against *L. australis, L. icterohaemorrhagiae, L. autumnalis*, and *L. Pomona*. In their study maximum activity was reported against *L. australis, L. icterohaemorrhagiae* with an MIC value of 200 200µg/ml concentration [60].

The chloroform extract of *Piper betle L.* leaf exhibited anti leptospiral activity. The MIC (minimum inhibitory concentration) was in the range of 17.5 to 500µg/ml for the serovars *L. australis* and *L. patoc*. The MLC(Minimum leptospirocidal concentration) 200-600 500µg/ml. The disruptive effect of crude compound of the chloroform extract of *Piper betle* on *Leptospira australis* cell membrane was assessed by using phyto chemical mediated propidium iodide uptake. Among the serovars, the *L. autumnalis, L. javanica, L. sejroe L. icterohaemorrhagiae*, and *L. patoc* were found to be the most susceptible to chloroform extract of *Piper betle* compared with other serovars included in this study. The increased uptake of propidium iodide in the *P. betle* extract-treated cells of *L. interrogans*, further confirmed the earlier findings that the phytochemical in *piper betel* alters the cell membrane structure, resulting in the disruption of the permeability barrier of microbial membrane structures. This may be the reason for its anti leptosiral action [61].

The crude extracts from *Garcinia mangostana* exhibited activity both non-pathogenic and pathogenic leptospira. The purified xanthones from *G. mangostana* and penicillin G for a non-pathogenic (*L. biflexa* serovar Patoc) and pathogenic (*L. interrogans* serovar Bataviae, Autumnalis, Javanica and Saigon) leptospire showed syngestic effect. Xanthones from fruit pericarp of *G. mangostana* with significant antibacterial activity may be used to control leptospirosis. The combination of xanthone with antibiotic penicillin G enhances the antileptospiral efficacy [62]. The xanthone responsible for this activity is γ-mangostin.

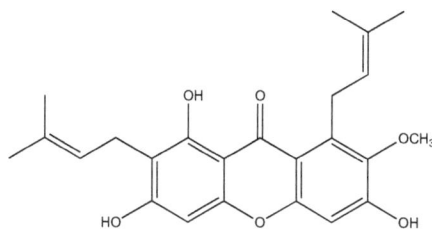

γ-mangostin

The anti-leptospiral potential of hexane, ethyl acetate, and methanol extracts of Zingiber zerumbet were studied. The hexane extract of Zingiber zerumbet showed significant antiletopira activity against *L. interrogans* serovar Canicola. IC 50 value was found to be 125 µg/ml towards *L. interrogans* serovar Australis, $IC_{25}$ value 15.63 µg/ml towards *L.* interrogans serovar Batavie, and $IC_{50}$ value 109 µg/ml towards *L. biflexa* serovar Patoc. However, ethyl acetate and methanol extracts exhibited a weak/mild anti-leptospiral activity [63].

*Adhatoda vasica* extracts exhibited anti leptospira activity against *L. interrogans*. MIC of the extracts was reported as 5mg/ml. this was comparable with activity of penicillin [64]. This herb is already used by traditional healers to cure liver disorders. The leaf of the *Adhatoda vasica* had been reported to contain Quinazoline Alkaloids (vasicine, N-oxides of vasicine, vasicinone, deoxyvasieine. oxyvasicinine malontone), and essential oil. The observed inhibition of Leptospira interrogans in the ethanolic extracts of *Adhatoda vasica* is close to the impact of penicillin. Besides the cellular break, inclusion bodies were also absent in the *Adhatoda vasica* treated *Leptospira interrogans* serovar Louisiana cells.

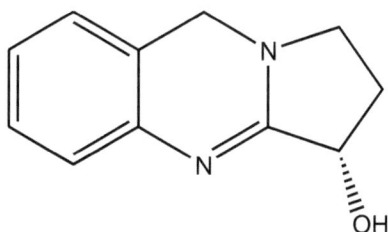

Vasicine

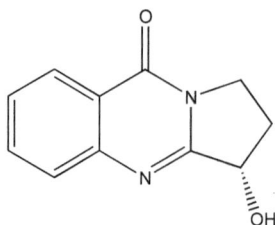

Vasicinone

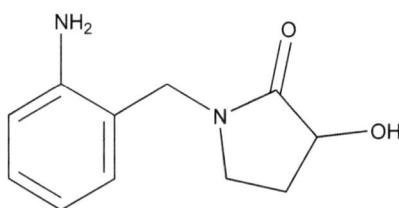

Vasicol

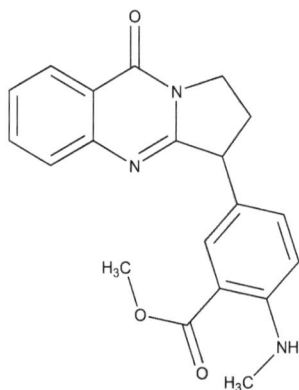

Anisitone

Leaves of plant *Boesenbergia rotunda* are used by Nicobarsee tribe of Andaman and Nicobar Islands, India to treat leptospirosis fever. The MIC of methanolic extract ranged between 62.5-125μg/ml in both micro dilution and macro dilution. The GC/MS analysis of methanol extracts enabled in identifying 25 components [65].

The Q. *infectoria* gall extract displays anti-microbial inhibition and killing activity against the pathogenic Leptospira isolates. The minimum inhibitory concentration (MIC) of aqueous Q. infectoria gall extract against the *L. interrogans* serovar Javanica and the *L. interrogans* serovar Icterohaemorrhagiae, at concentrations ranging from 4.00 mg/mL to 0.0078 mg/mL. Pyrogallol, a hydrolyzable tannin with three hydroxyl groups and alpha-beta double bonds is responsible for antimicrobial property [66].

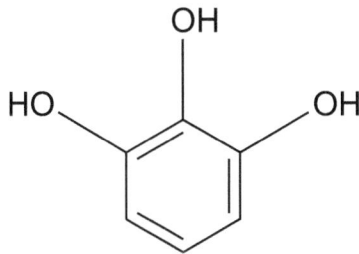

## Pyrogallol

K.S.Uma *et al.* in their study reported that the Siddha drugs Nilavembu kudineer and Seenthil sarkarai is having anti leptospiral activity but the drug Seenthil sarkarai was shown in lesser concentration of MIC compare to the drug Nilavembu kudineer for anti leptospiral activity [67].

The methanolic extract from leaves of Canarium odontophyllum has a potential to control leptospirosis. The IC50 value of methanol extract was 4.60 mg/mL and 2.25 mg/mL against serovar Bataviae and serovar Javanica, respectively. Both Leptospira used in this study which was *L. interrogans* serovar Bataviae and *L. borgpetersenii* serovar Javanica were confirmed pathogenic with the presence of band at756bp obtained with LipL32 based primers. Genomic DNA degradation was observed in L. borgpetersenii serovar Javanica but not in *L. interrogans* serovar Bataviae [68].

Siti *et al.* studied anti leptospiral properties of *Trigona thoracica* against pathogenic Leptospira species (spp.) and its synergistic effects with commonly prescribed antibiotics. Aqueous extract propolis (AEP) and ethanolic extracts propolis (EEP) were used. p. The synergy result showed that only a combination of AEP and penicillin G against serovar Australis has demonstrated a synergistic effect with the FIC index of 0.38. Morphological study using SEM showed significant structural changes of the treated Leptospira spp [69].

## SYNTHETIC ANALOGS FOR THE TREATMENT OF LEPTOSPIROSIS

A series of 6,7-dihydro-3H-pyrano[4,3-c]isoxazol-3-one derivatives were synthesized by Ilangovan *et al.*, *in vivo* and *in vitro* antileptospiral studies were reported. The MIC for the synthesized compounds were in the range of 62.5-500 µg/mL. The five compounds such as 10b, 10d, 10f, 10g, and 10j showed inhibition at lower concentration of 250 µg/mL itself. The structure activity relationship of compounds shows that substituent at 4th position of pyrano isaxazolone has an important influence on the activity against leptospiral serovars, and the compound 10g with a thienyl substituent is a potential lead for further study [70].

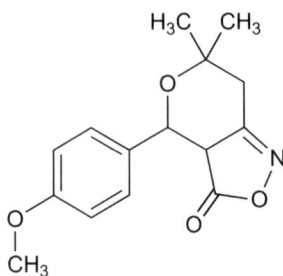

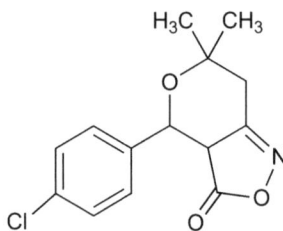

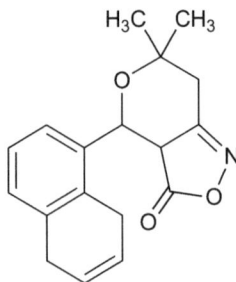

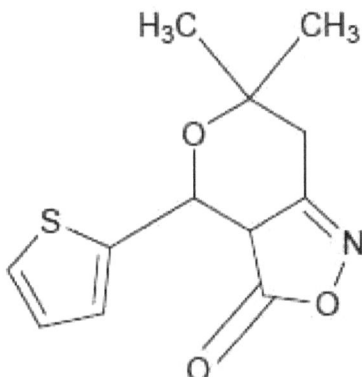

Five azomethines of aryl oxazole were synthesized by Niraimathi *et al.,* [71].The research reported the *in vitro* screening for leptospirosis. Among the 5 compounds compound 7C was found to be effective at low concentration. It showed arrest in the motility of the organism at the concentration of 500μgm/mL. This compound had 4-chlorophenyl substitution.

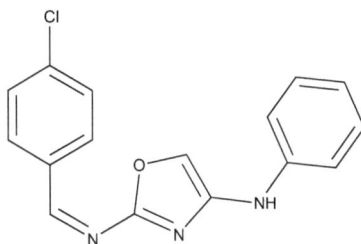

7C

Puratchikody *et al.,* had reported a simple and efficient method has been developed for the synthesis of series of N-Mannich bases of (E)-3-(phenylimino/4-chlorophenylimino)-2,3-dihydro-1-[(N-substituted piperazinyl) methyl]quinox-aline-2-(1H)-one 4a-f and 5a-f. [70]. All the synthesized compounds were screened for *in vitro* leptospirocidal activty against Leptospira *interrogans*. The potent compounds 5a, 5b and 5c with ciprofloxacin, norfloxacin, and sparfloxacin showed maximum activity during *in vitro* studies were subjected to *in vivo* studies. The inhibitory activity of enzymes carboxypeptidase and transpeptidase, in leptospirosis by the synthesized compounds were determined. 3D-QSAR studies model developed showed the need for more hydrophobic and less steric groups as substituent groups to enhance the *in vitro* activity [72].

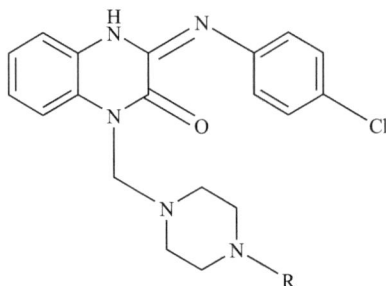

Synthesis of a new (E)-3-(4-or3-Aminophenylimino) quinoxaline-2(3H)-one oxime Schiff base derivatives and evaluation of the anti-leptospiral activity against Leptospira *icterohaemorrhagiae* was reported by C.Gopi *et al.,* [73] The structural activity relationship study suggests that 2, 3 di-substituted quinoxaline and its derivatives are needed for anti-leptospiral activity. Compounds bearing with an electron attracting substitutes on phenyl ring were exhibiting better activity against spirochete bacteria. Compounds 6c and 5c were constituted with the nitro group at the meta position of phenyl ring had considered as lead compounds and exhibited significant activity. Compound 5e and 6e have been constituted with a carboxylic acid on phenyl ring had been shown very excellent activity against *Leptospira icterohaemorrhagiae* strain as compared to penicillin G. Two more compound 5b and 6b showed an interesting activity against spirochete bacteria. Whereas, the compound substituted with an electron-donating group or un substituted on the phenyl ring offered a very low activity against *Leptospira icterohaemorrhagiae*. Compounds 5d and 6d possessed an attachment of $OCH_3$ and OH groups on phenyl ring had shown the least effect on spirochete bacteria. Compounds 5a and 6a have been constituted with un substituted phenyl ring had shown very negligible response against spirochetes as compared to penicillin G. In addition to that hydroxylated compound (5f and 6f) at the para position of phenyl ring had been shown remarkable activity against *Leptospira icterohaemorrhagia* as compared to penicillin G.

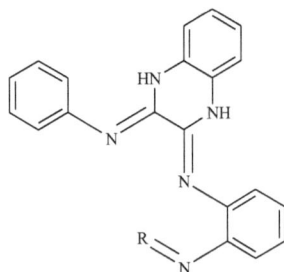

Ten new Quinoxaline bearing Azetidinone were synthesized by cyclo-condensation of Schiff bases of Quinoxaline-2,3-dione and tested. *In vitro* Leptospirocidal activity of the synthesized compounds was scrutinized using cultures of *Leptospira icterohaemorrhagiae* in EMJH medium at 37°C. It was concluded that among the synthesized compounds hydroxyl-substituted compounds and methoxy substituted compounds shows a high percentage of inhibition against the tested micro-organisms compared to standard drug Benzyl Penicillin [74].

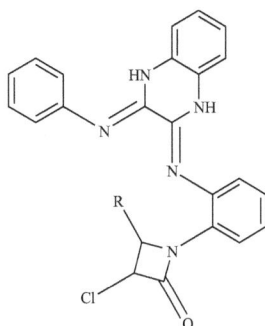

Chandan Shivamallu reported the antileptospiral activity of peptide- containing indole ring [75]. They reported the synthesis of a novel class of pseudo-peptides derived by coupling an amino acid with a heterocyclic moiety containing a free amine group using suitable coupling agents. The compound 4c has shown the best activity at 25, 50, and 75 g/mL, whereas other two compounds have also shown activity but, less when compared to 4c.

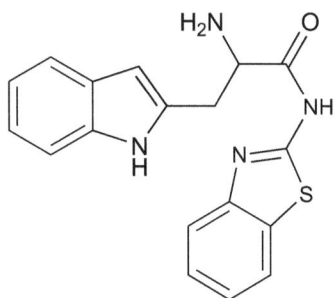

4a

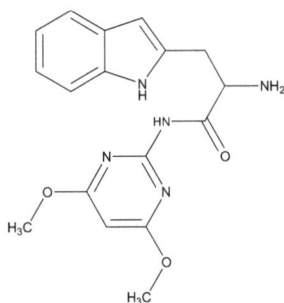

4b

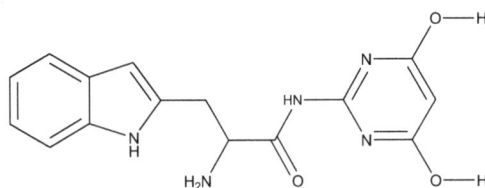

4c

## BIOCHEMICAL PARAMETERS

Micronutrients such as iron, calcium, and magnesium may be associated with leptospirosis. Iron is required for the growth of leptospires. They are very sensitive to the presence of iron chelators and also to low iron levels [76]. *Leptospira* infection may influence iron absorption and metabolism and circulating micronutrient concentrations. Increased serum ferritin concentrations may be attributable to the acute phase response to infection [77].

During leptospirosis infection, there are hemorrhages at mucous membranes, peritoneum, muscles, and organs such as kidneys and lungs [78]. Leptospira-infected macrophages had significantly elevated $Ca^{2+}$ concentrations, apoptosis, and necrosis compared to uninfected cells. Increased calcium level suggests that leptospirosis infection is in progress. Hypomagnesaemia is associated with pathogen infection [79]. The infection leads to the excretion of more potassium due to tubular dysfunction. This leads to low potassium levels and sodium levels in the blood [80]. Abnormal Serum Amylase and lipase levels are reported  during infection. AST increased in 95% of patients. Proteinuria is present in leptospirosis due to mild alteration in the glomerulus during the infection.

Biochemical parameters involved were serum total cholesterol, serum HDL-cholesterol, serum creatinine, serum urea, serum glutamate pyruvate transaminase (SGPT), serum glutamate oxaloacetate transaminase (SGOT), total bilirubin, and triglycerides. During the infection, all these parameters were elevated in serum. The increase in serum creatinine level during leptospirosis was due to stimulation of the enzyme nitric oxide synthase which produced more nitric oxide which leads to an increase in serum creatinine level while the infection caused renal damage due to which serum urea level was increased. Stimulation of serum lipase and triglyceride synthase in leptospirosis elevated the triglyceride level. The increase in bilirubin level was due to excessive hemolysis. During infection, RBC and platelet counts were decreased while ESR and WBC counts were elevated. The administration of test compounds increased the RBC and platelet counts and reduced the WBC and ESR counts. The infection with leptospirosis caused excessive hemolysis which reduced RBC and platelet counts. On the other hand, WBC count and ESR were increased in leptospirosis. Administration of test compounds decreased the elevated levels of WBC and ESR. In contrast, there was an increase in RBC and platelet counts after administrations of test compounds.

## HISTOPATHOLOGICAL CHANGES IN LEPTOSPIROSIS

Many histopathological changes were observed with leptospiral infection. During hematoxylin-eosin (H-E) staining kidneys of infected rats showed many changes. Interstitial nephritis was the most common lesion. It showed inflammatory infiltrate with lymphoplasmacytic cells and histocytes. Focal compromise in peri vascular location was observed [81]. Cystic dilation of tubules, glomerular atrophy, multifocal interstitial mononuclear infiltration, and neutrophilic infiltration were reported in infected dogs. Lymphoplasmacytic and neutrophilic tubulointerstitial nephritis were also reported [82].

Congestion of the sinusoids, varying degrees of degenerative changes, and bile duct hyperplasia with focal to multifocal areas of mononuclear cell infiltrations and periportal cirrhosis were reported in the liver of dog. Hepatocyte dissociation with intrahepatic cholestasis and hepatocytic necrosis were the hallmarks of leptospiral infection in dogs [83].

Septal congestion, multifocal alveolar hemorrhage, and edema, occasionally with focal fibrin exudation were reported in histopathology of lungs during leptospirosis infection. A recent work by Del Carlo Bernardi *et al.,* found, in vessels of human lungs in leptospirotic patients dying of hemorrhagic pneumopathy, an increased expression of intercellular adhesion molecule, vascular adhesion molecule, and Toll-like receptor, compared with the normal lung [84]. Leptospirosis exhibits well-known alterations of aquaporin 1 which has a role in regulating the vascular permeability to water in the lung [85]. This resulted in alveolar edema [86].

## *IN SILICO* STUDIES FOR LEPTOSPIRAL DRUGS

Nair Vandana P. *et al*. have carried out docking studies using software tools like Accelrys Biosolve-IT FlexX and Gold 5.1 to investigate the binding affinity of 50 natural and 50 synthetic compounds with human p38α mitogen activated protein kinases. The docking study concluded that natural compounds aodium curcuminate and curcumin which belong to same family of *curcuma longa* as well as Gemichalcone_B are the probable compounds for leptospirosis [87].

The outer membrane lipoprotein "LipL32" is expressed in pathogenic leptospira. The binding interaction of doxycycline with LipL32 was reported by sandeep Solomon *et al*. The results revealed that the potent antigenic site for the LipL32 protein of pathogenic leptospiral species was located between 18th to 27th amino acid residues and 93rd to 105th amino acid residues of the LipL32 protein. The docking results revealed that doxycycline is exhibiting docking with LipL32 proteins of Leptospira with the same pharmacoporic site located at 21st Alanine (hydrophobic), 22nd Phenylalanine (very hydrophobic) and 23rd Glycine, (amphiphilic) amino acids, respectively [88].

A data-set of BB-78485 structural analogs were docked with LpxC in Maestro v9.2 virtual screening workflow by Dibyabhaba Pradhan *et al.,* [89]. This research has identified 12 compounds as potential inhibitors of LpxC. Para-(benzoyl--phenylalanine - that showed the lowest XP Gscore (-10.35 kcal/mol) - was predicted to have the best binding affinity towards LpxC.

Gupta and Sahu have carried out docking of 308 natural antibacterial and 144 natural antiviral phytochemicals against Peptide deformylase, which is an important enzyme needed for the survival of leptospiral bacteria. The active site calculated with 530.6 A area and 978 A of volume and consisted of the following amino acid residues. ALA (A) 44, GLU (A) 45, GLY (A) 46, VAL (A) 47, GLY (A) 48, GLN (A) 53, ARG (A) 70, TYR (A) 71, THR (A) 74, PHE (A) 97, TRP (A) 98, GLU (A) 99, GLY (A) 100, CYS (A) 101, LEU (A) 102, VAL (A) 104, PRO (A) 105, GLY (A) 106, MET (A) 107, ARG (A) 107, TYR (A) 136, ILE (A) 139, VAL (A) 140, HIS (A) 143, GLU (A) 144, ASN (A) 166. Among the antibacterial phytochemical Betulinic-Acid, Glycyrrhetinic-Acid, Oxyasiaticoside, Tomatine and Ursolic Acid exhibited better binding affinity with enzyme.

Saikosaponin-A, Betulin and Bilobetin has exhibited the optimum binding affinity among antiviral compounds [90].

T.H. Samaha has reported the binding interaction of the protein with the plasma membrane phosphoinositides (PIP). This research reported binding energies of -14.04 and -11.64 kcal/mol respectively for PIP2 and PIP3 interaction [91].

## BIOMARKERS IN LEPTOSPIROSIS

Various studies have shown that cytokines and serum proteins are promising biomarkers for leptospirosis severity. TNF α is a cytokinin that plays a major role in vasodilation, tissue development and death, cell differentiation and immune-mediated disease Estavoyer *et al.*, reported the high TNF α levels in non-fatal leptospirosis [92]. High level of TNF-α was associated with higher mortality seen in patients suffering from severe leptospirosis. Interleukin10 (IL-10) is another important cytokine involved in the leptospirosis severity. IL-6 is an independent predictor of death in leptospirosis as suggested by Reis *et al.,* [93]. A high expression of chemokines CXCL1/KC, CXCL2/MIP-2, CCL5/RANTES is also reported in this disease [94]. Xue Ting Tan reported the expression of apolipoprotein A-I (APOA-I), serum amyloid A (SAA), transferrin (TF), haptoglobin, (HP) and transthyretin (TTR) in mild and severe leptospirosis [95]. Rajneesh Srivastava reported 6 significant proteins in leptospirosis. Among 6 proteins, 4 proteins namely Apolipoprotein A1 precursor, serum albumin precursor, Apolipoprotein A 1V precursor, complement C4 precursor were downregulated and 2 proteins alpha 1 antitrypsin precursor and alpha 1 B glycoprotein precursor were down regulated [96]. α-1-antitrypsin, vitronectin, ceruloplasmin, G-protein signaling regulator, apolipoprotein A-I were reported as biomarkers by Srivastava *et al.*

Charles Solomon Akino Mercy identified circulating miRNAs as authentic biomarkers for early diagnosis of leptospirosis. miRNAs are 22-nucleotide-long small noncoding regulatory RNA molecules that regulate gene expression post transcriptional through complementary base pairing with thousands of messenger RNAs and play important roles in regulating diverse physiological, developmental, and pathophysiological processes. Analysis of the miRNA profile of the extracellular media of control and TLR2 knockdown cells with or without LPS treatment showed ~18 miRNAs to be upregulated (>10-fold) in THP1 cells treated with LPS compared to untreated controls, whereas knocking down TLR2 normalized the upregulated miRNA levels, indicating that these miRNAs are specific to the TLR2-LPS immune axis and thus can serve as biomarkers [97].

## PREVENTION AND CONTROL

### Personal protection

Avoidance of contact with contaminated water or mud. Workers in flooded fields must be advised to use rubber shoes and gloves.

### Health education

The main step in preventing the spread of infection is creating awareness about diseases and prevention.

### Chemoprophylaxis

During the peak transmission season, Doxycycline 200 mg, once a week, maybe given to vulnerable people.

### Rodent control

Rodents are the reservoirs of *leptospira interogans*. Four species of rodents, *Rattusrattus* (House rat), *Rattus norvegicus* (Norway rat), *Bandicota bengalensis* (Lesser bandicoot) and *Bandicota indica* (Larger bandicoot) are so far found to be reservoirs for this bacterium in India. Hence controlling these reservoir species with proper strategic planning and management will reduce the incidence of the disease in the affected areas.

### Mapping of water bodies for establishing a proper drainage system

Mapping of water bodies for establishing a proper drainage system must be carried out.

### Vaccination of animals

Leptospiral vaccines confer a limited duration of immunity. Boosters are needed every one to two years. Vaccination should however be very selective and used only in endemic situations having a high incidence of leptospirosis. The vaccine must contain the dominant local serovars.

## CONCLUSION

From the detailed literature review carried out, it was found that only very few synthetic derivatives are reported for leptospirosis. Though many natural products are reported for leptospirosis, they lack molecular mechanisms. The available drugs for the treatment of this disease also have a side effect. So there is a need to develop more synthetic compounds for treating leptospirosis.

From this literature review, we came to know that many drug targets are reported for leptospirosis. So, future researchers can design some synthetic analogs, and can carry out docking studies with any one of the reported drug targets, estimate the binding energy and then synthesize the compounds with high binding energy.

## CONSENT FOR PUBLICATION

Not applicable.

## CONFLICT OF INTEREST

The authors declare no conflict of interest, financial or otherwise.

## ACKNOWLEDGEMENT

Declared none.

## REFERENCES

[1]    Dunay S, Bass J, Stremick J. Leptospirosis: a global health burden in review. Emerg Med (Los Angel) 2016; 6(336): 2.
[http://dx.doi.org/10.4172/2165-7548.1000336]

[2]    Terpstra WJ. Historical perspectives in leptospirosis. Indian J Med Microbiol 2006; 24(4): 316-20.
[http://dx.doi.org/10.1016/S0255-0857(21)02309-4] [PMID: 17185865]

[3]    Dikken H, Kmety E. Serological typing methods of leptospires. Methods Microbiol 1978; 11: 260-95.
[http://dx.doi.org/10.1016/S0580-9517(08)70493-8]

[4]    Schüffner WA. The present state of the leptospira question. Nederlands Tijdschrift voor Geneeskunde. 1928; 13.

[5]    Kuenen WA. Demonstration of the spirochaete ictero-haemorrhagica found in Japan (with Weil's disease). *In: Proceedings of a meeting of the Netherlands Society for Tropical Medicine.* Ned Tijdschr Geneeskd 1917; 10: 902-26.

[6]    Alston JM, Broom JC, Doughty CJA. Leptospirosis in man and animals. Edinburgh: Livingstone 1958.(5):

[7]    Oaks SC Jr, Shope RE, Lederberg J, Eds. Emerging infections: microbial threats to health in the United States. National Academies Press 1992.

[8]    Michin NA, Azinow SA. Spirochaetal jaundice of cattle in North Caucasus (translated title). Sovyet Vet 1935; 10: 23-7.

[9]    Ellis WA. . InLeptospira and leptospirosis Springer 2015; pp. 99-137.
[http://dx.doi.org/10.1007/978-3-662-45059-8_6]

[10]    Christopher GW, Agan MB, Cieslak TJ, Olson PE. History of U.S. military contributions to the study of bacterial zoonoses. Mil Med 2005; 170(4) (Suppl.): 39-48.
[http://dx.doi.org/10.7205/MILMED.170.4S.39] [PMID: 15916282]

[11]    Gochenour WS Jr, Smadel JE, Jackson EB, Evans LB, Yager RH. Leptospiral etiology of Fort Bragg

fever. Public Health Rep 1952; 67(8): 811-3.
[http://dx.doi.org/10.2307/4588208] [PMID: 12983521]

[12]    Gale NB, Alexander AD, Evans LB, Yager RH, Matheney RG. An outbreak of leptospirosis among U. S. army troops in the Canal Zone. Am J Trop Med Hyg 1966; 15(1): 64-70.
[http://dx.doi.org/10.4269/ajtmh.1966.15.64] [PMID: 5902111]

[13]    Corwin A, Ryan A, Bloys W, Thomas R, Deniega B, Watts D. A waterborne outbreak of leptospirosis among United States military personnel in Okinawa, Japan. Int J Epidemiol 1990; 19(3): 743-8.
[http://dx.doi.org/10.1093/ije/19.3.743] [PMID: 2262273]

[14]    https://www.thehindu.com/news/cities/Kochi/spike-in-leptospirosis-cases-in-ernakulam-w-rries-health-authorities/article32651177.ece

[15]    World Health Organization. Leptospirosis worldwide, 1999. Weekly Epidemiological Record= Relevé épidémiologique hebdomadaire 1999; 74(29): 237-42.

[16]    Michel V, Branger C, Andre-Fontaine G. Epidemiology of leptospirosis. Rev Cubana Med Trop 2002; 54(1): 7-10.
[PMID: 15846932]

[17]    Costa F, Hagan JE, Calcagno J, *et al.* Global morbidity and mortality of leptospirosis: a systematic review. PLoS Negl Trop Dis 2015; 9(9): e0003898.
[http://dx.doi.org/10.1371/journal.pntd.0003898] [PMID: 26379143]

[18]    Picardeau M. Diagnosis and epidemiology of leptospirosis. Med Mal Infect 2013; 43(1): 1-9.
[http://dx.doi.org/10.1016/j.medmal.2012.11.005] [PMID: 23337900]

[19]    Himani D, Suman MK, Mane BG. Epidemiology of leptospirosis: an Indian perspective. J Foodborne Zoonotic Dis 2013; 1(1): 6-13.

[20]    Colavita G, Paoletti M. [Leptospirosis: occupational risk in the chain of food of animal origin]. G Ital Med Lav Ergon 2007; 29(1): 21-4.
[PMID: 17569414]

[21]    Damude DF, Jones CJ, White HS, Myers DM. The problem of human leptospirosis in Barbados. Trans R Soc Trop Med Hyg 1979; 73(2): 169-77.
[http://dx.doi.org/10.1016/0035-9203(79)90202-5] [PMID: 473305]

[22]    Cacciapuoti B, Nuti M, Pinto A, Sabrie AM. Human leptospirosis in Somalia: a serological survey. Trans R Soc Trop Med Hyg 1982; 76(2): 178-82.
[http://dx.doi.org/10.1016/0035-9203(82)90270-X] [PMID: 6980503]

[23]    Ratnam S, Sundararaj T, Thyagarajan SP, Rao RS, Madanagopalan N, Subramanian S. Serological evidence of leptospirosis in jaundice and pyrexia of unknown origin. Indian J Med Res 1983; 77: 427-30.
[PMID: 6874030]

[24]    Ratnam S, Sundararaj T, Subramanian S. Serological evidence of leptospirosis in a human population following an outbreak of the disease in cattle. Trans R Soc Trop Med Hyg 1983; 77(1): 94-8.
[http://dx.doi.org/10.1016/0035-9203(83)90027-5] [PMID: 6679368]

[25]    Ahmed IP. Serological studies on leptospirosis in Pakistan. J Pak Med Assoc 1987; 37(9): 233-6.
[PMID: 3119890]

[26]    Everard CO, Hayes RJ, Edwards CN. Leptospiral infection in school-children from Trinidad and Barbados. Epidemiol Infect 1989; 103(1): 143-56.
[http://dx.doi.org/10.1017/S0950268800030442] [PMID: 2789146]

[27]    Muthusethupathi MA, Shivakumar S. Acute renal failure due to leptospirosis. J Assoc Physicians India 1987; 35(9): 631-3.
[PMID: 3436932]

[28]    Sehgal SC, Murhekar MV, Sugunan AP. Outbreak of leptospirosis with pulmonary involvement in

north Andaman. Indian J Med Res 1995; 102: 9-12.
[PMID: 7558211]

[29]   Outbreak of acute febrile illness among athletes participating in triathlons--Wisconsin and Illinois, 1998. MMWR Morb Mortal Wkly Rep 1998; 47(28): 585-8.
[PMID: 9694638]

[30]   Mohammed H, Nozha C, Hakim K, Abdelaziz F, Rekia B. Leptospira: morphology, classification and pathogenesis. J Bacteriol Parasitol 2011; 2(06)
[http://dx.doi.org/10.4172/2155-9597.1000120]

[31]   Shaked Y, Shpilberg O, Samra D, Samra Y. Leptospirosis in pregnancy and its effect on the fetus: case report and review. Clin Infect Dis 1993; 17(2): 241-3.
[http://dx.doi.org/10.1093/clinids/17.2.241] [PMID: 8399874]

[32]   Ellinghausen HC Jr. The effect of aeration upon the growth of leptospira serotypes. Am J Vet Res 1966; 27(119): 975-9.
[PMID: 5338548]

[33]   Daher EF, Lima RS, Silva Júnior GB, *et al*. Clinical presentation of leptospirosis: a retrospective study of 201 patients in a metropolitan city of Brazil. Braz J Infect Dis 2010; 14(1): 3-10.
[http://dx.doi.org/10.1016/S1413-8670(10)70002-7] [PMID: 20428646]

[34]   Haake DA, Levett PN. Leptospirosis in humans InLeptospira and leptospirosis 2015 . Berlin, Heidelberg: Springer 2015; pp. 65-97.

[35]   Amineni U, Pradhan D, Marisetty H. In silico identification of common putative drug targets in Leptospira *interrogans*. J Chem Biol 2010; 3(4): 165-73.
[http://dx.doi.org/10.1007/s12154-010-0039-1] [PMID: 21572503]

[36]   Gupta R, Verma R, Pradhan D, Jain AK, Umamaheswari A, Rai CS. An in silico approach towards identification of novel drug targets in pathogenic species of Leptospira. PLoS One 2019; 14(8): e0221446.
[http://dx.doi.org/10.1371/journal.pone.0221446] [PMID: 31430340]

[37]   Lata KS, Kumar S, Vaghasia V, *et al*. Exploring Leptospiral proteomes to identify potential candidates for vaccine design against Leptospirosis using an immunoinformatics approach. Sci Rep 2018; 8(1): 6935.
[http://dx.doi.org/10.1038/s41598-018-25281-3] [PMID: 29720698]

[38]   Lata KS, Kumar S, Vaghasia V. *et al*. Exploring Leptospiral proteomes to identify potential candidates for vaccine design against Leptospirosis using an immunoinformatics approach. Sci Rep 2018; 8: 6935.
[http://dx.doi.org/10.1038/s41598-018-25281-3]

[39]   Vernel-Pauillac F, Werts C. Recent findings related to immune responses against leptospirosis and novel strategies to prevent infection. Microbes Infect 2018; 20(9-10): 578-88.
[http://dx.doi.org/10.1016/j.micinf.2018.02.001] [PMID: 29452258]

[40]   Snow Setzer M, Sharifi-Rad J, Setzer WN. The search for herbal antibiotics: An *in-silico* investigation of antibacterial phytochemicals. Antibiotics (Basel) 2016; 5(3): 30.
[http://dx.doi.org/10.3390/antibiotics5030030] [PMID: 27626453]

[41]   Barb AW, Zhou P. Mechanism and inhibition of LpxC: an essential zinc-dependent deacetylase of bacterial lipid A synthesis. Curr Pharm Biotechnol 2008; 9(1): 9-15.
[http://dx.doi.org/10.2174/138920108783497668] [PMID: 18289052]

[42]   https://www.rcsb.org/structure/4U06

[43]   Georrge JJ. A bioinformatics approach for the identification of potential drug targets and identification of drug-like molecules for ribosomal protein L6 of staphylococcus species. In: Proceedings of 9th National Level Science Symposium on Recent Trends in Science and Technology. 320-7.

[44] Zuerner R, Haake D, Adler B, Segers R. Technological advances in the molecular biology of Leptospira. 2000; 2(4): 455-62.

[45] Solmon KS, Suneetha G, Kiranmayi P, Reddy IB. Docking studies of doxycycline on pathogenic Leptospira Species with common pharmacopore. International journal of advanced research in science and technology. (1): 5-9.

[46] Cumberland P, Everard CO, Levett PN. Assessment of the efficacy of an IgM-elisa and microscopic agglutination test (MAT) in the diagnosis of acute leptospirosis. Am J Trop Med Hyg 1999; 61(5): 731-4.
[http://dx.doi.org/10.4269/ajtmh.1999.61.731] [PMID: 10586903]

[47] Cui JJ, Xiao GX, Chen TZ, *et al.* Further evaluation of one-point microcapsule agglutination test for diagnosis of leptospirosis. Epidemiol Infect 1991; 106(3): 561-5.
[http://dx.doi.org/10.1017/S0950268800067625] [PMID: 2050209]

[48] Silva MV. Dot-ELISA-IgM in saliva for the diagnosis of human leptospirosis using polyester fabric-resin as support (preliminary report). Rev. Inst. Med. trop. S. Paulo 1994; (Oct): 475-8.

[49] Levett PN, Branch SL, Whittington CU, Edwards CN, Paxton H. Two methods for rapid serological diagnosis of acute leptospirosis. Clin Diagn Lab Immunol 2001; 8(2): 349-51.
[http://dx.doi.org/10.1128/CDLI.8.2.349-351.2001] [PMID: 11238220]

[50] Budihal SV, Perwez K. Leptospirosis diagnosis: competancy of various laboratory tests. J Clin Diagn Res 2014; 8(1): 199-202.
[http://dx.doi.org/10.7860/JCDR/2014/6593.3950] [PMID: 24596774]

[51] Xiao X, Wu ZC, Chou KC. A multi-label classifier for predicting the subcellular localization of gram-negative bacterial proteins with both single and multiple sites. PLoS One 2011; 6(6): e20592.
[http://dx.doi.org/10.1371/journal.pone.0020592] [PMID: 21698097]

[52] Pinne M, Haake D. Immuno-fluorescence assay of leptospiral surface-exposed proteins. J Vis Exp 2011; (53): e2805.
[PMID: 21750491]

[53] Guerreiro H, Croda J, Flannery B, *et al.* Leptospiral proteins recognized during the humoral immune response to leptospirosis in humans. Infect Immun 2001; 69(8): 4958-68.
[http://dx.doi.org/10.1128/IAI.69.8.4958-4968.2001] [PMID: 11447174]

[54] Banfi E, Cinco M, Delia S, *et al.* New trends in the rapid serodiagnosis of leptospirosis. Zentralbl Bakteriol Mikrobiol Hyg A 1984; 257(4): 503-7.
[http://dx.doi.org/10.1016/S0176-6724(84)80071-1] [PMID: 6506922]

[55] Millar BD, Chappel RJ, Adler B. Detection of leptospires in biological fluids using DNA hybridisation. Vet Microbiol 1987; 15(1-2): 71-8.
[http://dx.doi.org/10.1016/0378-1135(87)90131-3] [PMID: 3439017]

[56] Terpstra WJ. Typing leptospira from the perspective of a reference laboratory. Acta Leiden 1992; 60(2): 79-87.
[PMID: 1485498]

[57] Chander MP, Kumar KV, Shriram AN, Vijayachari P. Anti-leptospiral activities of an endemic plant Glyptopetalum calocarpum (Kurz.) Prain used as a medicinal plant by Nicobarese of Andaman and Nicobar Islands. Nat Prod Res 2015; 29(16): 1575-7.
[http://dx.doi.org/10.1080/14786419.2014.985679] [PMID: 25482276]

[58] Prabhu N, Innocent JP, Chinnaswamy P, Natarajaseenivasan K, Sarayu L. *in vitro* Evaluation of Eclipta alba against Serogroups of Leptospira *interrogans* Indian J Pharm Sci 2008; 70(6): 788-91.
[http://dx.doi.org/10.4103/0250-474X.49124] [PMID: 21369443]

[59] Chandan S, Umesha S, Balamurugan V. Antileptospiral, antioxidant and DNA damaging properties of *Eclipta alba* and *Phyllanthus amarus*. Sci Rep 2012; 1: 231.

[60]    Natarajaseenivasan K.*in vitro* anti leptospiral activity of ethanolic extract of the leaf of Andrographis paniculata Nees (Acanthaceae). Int J Curr Res Biol Med 2017; 2(2): 24-7.
[http://dx.doi.org/10.22192/ijcrbm.2017.02.02.004]

[61]    Begum SN. 2016; Ethnobotanicals of the western ghats. ethnobotany of india. 107.

[62]    Seesom W, Jaratrungtawee A, Suksamrarn S, Mekseepralard C, Ratananukul P, Sukhumsirichart W. Antileptospiral activity of xanthones from Garcinia mangostana and synergy of gamma-mangostin with penicillin G. BMC Complement Altern Med 2013; 13(1): 182-4.
[http://dx.doi.org/10.1186/1472-6882-13-182] [PMID: 23866810]

[63]    Hamid A, Abdul Aziz NA, Ibrahim L, Ibrahim FW, Jufri NF. Anti-leptospiral potential of Zingiber zerumbet (L.) Smith crude extracts against Leptospira spp. Front Pharmacol Conference Abstract: International Conference on Drug Discovery and Translational Medicine 2018 (ICDDTM '18) "Seizing Opportunities and Addressing Challenges of Precision Medicine.
[http://dx.doi.org/10.3389/conf.fphar.2018.63.00117]

[64]    Nelson J, Chairman K, Singh AR, Padmalatha C, Hepsibah B. Cytomorphological changes and inhibition of inclusion body formation in Leptospira *interrogans* on treatment with the extracts of *Adhatoda vasica*. Adv Tech Bio Med 2013; 1(1): 1-4.
[http://dx.doi.org/10.4172/2379-1764.1000101]

[65]    Chander MP, Vinod Kumar K, Lall C, Vimal Raj R, Vijayachari P. GC/MS profiling, *in vitro* anti-leptospiral and haemolytic activities of *Boesenbergia rotunda* (L.) Mansf. used as a medicinal plant by Nicobarese of Andaman and Nicobar Islands. Nat Prod Res 2016; 30(10): 1190-2.
[http://dx.doi.org/10.1080/14786419.2015.1046068] [PMID: 26114982]

[66]    Mustafa H, Ismail N, Wahab WNAWA. Anti-microbial activity of aqueous *Quercus infectoria* gall extract against pathogenic *Leptospira*. Malays J Med Sci 2018; 25(4): 42-50.
[http://dx.doi.org/10.21315/mjms2018.25.4.4] [PMID: 30914846]

[67]    Uma KS, Jacob M, Arumugam GA, Kalpana S, Natarajan M. *In vitro* antimicrobial activity of the siddha drugs seenthil sarkarai and nilavembu kudineer against leptospira. Int J Pharm Pharm Sci 2012; 4 (Suppl. 2): 75-8.

[68]    Ishak SA, Ariffudin S, Azmi FF, Hamid A, Ibrahim L, Basri DF. *In-vitro* antileptospiral activity of Canarium odontophyllum Miq. (Dabai) leaves extract. Malays J Microbiol 2019; 15(3): 1-6.

[69]    Ismail SR, Ismail S, Deris ZZ, Ismail N. *in vitro* Antileptospiral Activity of *Trigona thoracia* Propolis and its Synergistic Effects with Commonly Prescribed Antibiotics. Int Med J Malays 2020; 19(1): 1317.
[http://dx.doi.org/10.31436/imjm.v19i1.1317]

[70]    Ilangovan A, Sakthivel P, Sivasankari K, Mercy CS, Natarajaseenivasan K. Discovery of 6,7-dihydr--3H-pyrano[4,3-c]isoxazol-3-ones as a new class of pathogen specific anti-leptospiral agents. Eur J Med Chem 2017; 125: 29-40.
[http://dx.doi.org/10.1016/j.ejmech.2016.09.020] [PMID: 27643561]

[71]    Niraimathi V, Suresh AJ, Sriram L, Latha T. Antimicrobial study (*in vitro*) of azomethines of Aryl oxazoles. J Pharm Res 2011; 10(2): 83-4.

[72]    Puratchikody A, Natarajan R, Doble M, Iswarya SH, Vijayabharathi R. Synthesis, leptospirocidal activity and QSAR analysis of novel quinoxaline derivatives. Med Chem 2013; 9(2): 275-86.
[http://dx.doi.org/10.2174/1573406411309020010] [PMID: 22779788]

[73]    Gopi C, Sastry VG, Dhanaraju MD. Microwave-assisted synthesis, structural activity relationship and biological activity of some new quinoxaline Schiff base derivatives as highly potent spirochete bactericidal agents. Beni Suef Univ J Basic Appl Sci 2017; 6(1): 39-47.
[http://dx.doi.org/10.1016/j.bjbas.2016.12.007]

[74]    Natarajan R, Subramani A, Kesavan SK, Selvaraj D. Biological evaluation of some novel quinoxaline bearing azetidinones including leptospirocidal study. J Pharm Res 2013; 1: 775-80.

[75]   Shivamallu C, Sharanaiah U, Kollur SP, Mallesh NK, Hosakere RD, Balamurugan V. Pseudo-peptides as novel antileptospiral agents: synthesis and spectral characterization. Spectrochim Acta A Mol Biomol Spectrosc 2014; 118: 1152-7.
[http://dx.doi.org/10.1016/j.saa.2013.09.105] [PMID: 24184586]

[76]   Velineni S, Asuthkar S, Sritharan M. Iron limitation and expression of immunoreactive outer membrane proteins in Leptospira *interrogans* serovar icterohaemorrhagiae strain lai. Indian J Med Microbiol 2006; 24(4): 339-42.
[http://dx.doi.org/10.1016/S0255-0857(21)02316-1] [PMID: 17185872]

[77]   Herman HS, Mehta S, Cárdenas WB, Stewart-Ibarra AM, Finkelstein JL. Micronutrients and leptospirosis: a review of the current evidence. PLoS Negl Trop Dis 2016; 10(7): e0004652.
[http://dx.doi.org/10.1371/journal.pntd.0004652] [PMID: 27387046]

[78]   Vieira ML, de Andrade SA, Morais ZM, Vasconcellos SA, Dagli ML, Nascimento AL. Leptospira infection interferes with the prothrombinase complex assembly during experimental leptospirosis. Front Microbiol 2017; 8: 500.
[http://dx.doi.org/10.3389/fmicb.2017.00500] [PMID: 28400758]

[79]   Spichler A, Athanazio DA, Furtado J, Seguro A, Vinetz JM. Case report: severe, symptomatic hypomagnesemia in acute leptospirosis. Am J Trop Med Hyg 2008; 79(6): 915-7.
[http://dx.doi.org/10.4269/ajtmh.2008.79.915] [PMID: 19052304]

[80]   Baburaj P, Varma SS, Harikrishnan BL. Hypokalemic paralysis in leptospirosis. J Assoc Physicians India 2012; 60(3): 53-4.
[PMID: 22799118]

[81]   Sánchez MD, Cuervo J, Rave D, *et al.* Hereditary angioedema in Medellín (Colombia): Clinical evaluation and quality of life appraisal. Biomédica 2015; 35(3): 419-28.
[PMID: 26849703]

[82]   Birnbaum N, Barr SC, Center SA, Schermerhorn T, Randolph JF, Simpson KW. Naturally acquired leptospirosis in 36 dogs: serological and clinicopathological features. J Small Anim Pract 1998; 39(5): 231-6.
[http://dx.doi.org/10.1111/j.1748-5827.1998.tb03640.x] [PMID: 9631358]

[83]   Sessions JK, Greene CE. Canine leptospirosis: epidemiology, pathogenesis, and diagnosis. Compendium on continuing education for the practising veterinarian-north american edition 2004; 26(8): 606-24.

[84]   Del Carlo Bernardi F, Ctenas B, da Silva LF, *et al.* Immune receptors and adhesion molecules in human pulmonary leptospirosis. Hum Pathol 2012; 43(10): 1601-10.
[http://dx.doi.org/10.1016/j.humpath.2011.11.017] [PMID: 22436623]

[85]   Saadoun S, Papadopoulos MC, Hara-Chikuma M, Verkman AS. Impairment of angiogenesis and cell migration by targeted aquaporin-1 gene disruption. Nature 2005; 434(7034): 786-92.
[http://dx.doi.org/10.1038/nature03460] [PMID: 15815633]

[86]   De Brito T, Aiello VD, da Silva LF, *et al.* Human hemorrhagic pulmonary leptospirosis: pathological findings and pathophysiological correlations. PLoS One 2013; 8(8): e71743.
[http://dx.doi.org/10.1371/journal.pone.0071743] [PMID: 23951234]

[87]   Hamsa NS, Vivek C. Int. J. Drug Dev. & Res. Nair Vandana P1 2013.

[88]   Solmon KS, Suneetha G, Kiranmayi P, Reddy IB. Docking studies of doxycycline on pathogenic Leptospira Species with common pharmacopore. Int J Adv Res Sci Technol 2012; 1(1): 5-9.

[89]   Pradhan D, Priyadarshini V, Munikumar M, Swargam S, Umamaheswari A, Bitla A. Para-(benzoyl--phenylalanine as a potential inhibitor against LpxC of Leptospira spp.: homology modeling, docking, and molecular dynamics study. J Biomol Struct Dyn 2014; 32(2): 171-85.
[http://dx.doi.org/10.1080/07391102.2012.758056] [PMID: 23383626]

[90]  Gupta PK, Sahu B. Identification of natural compound inhibitors against peptide deformylase using virtual screening and molecular docking techniques. Bull Environ Pharmacol Life Sci 2015; 4: 70-80.

[91]  Samaha TH. Interactions of Leptospiral PI-PLC with the membrane phosphoinositides: an insight of the protein-phospholipid association in the pathogenesis. Int J Comput Biol Drug Des 2020; 13(2): 200-8.

[92]  Estavoyer JM, Racadot E, Couetdic G, Leroy J, Grosperrin L. Tumor necrosis factor in patients with leptospirosis. Reviews of infectious diseases 1991; 13(6): 1245-47.
[http://dx.doi.org/10.1093/clinids/13.6.1245]

[93]  Reis EA, Hagan JE, Ribeiro GS, *et al.* Cytokine response signatures in disease progression and development of severe clinical outcomes for leptospirosis. PLoS Negl Trop Dis 2013; 7(9): e2457.
[http://dx.doi.org/10.1371/journal.pntd.0002457] [PMID: 24069500]

[94]  Richer L, Potula HH, Melo R, Vieira A, Gomes-Solecki M. Mouse model for sublethal Leptospira *interrogans* infection. Infect Immun 2015; 83(12): 4693-700.
[http://dx.doi.org/10.1128/IAI.01115-15] [PMID: 26416909]

[95]  Tan XT, Amran FB, Thayan R, *et al.* Potential serum biomarkers associated with mild and severe leptospirosis infection: A cohort study in the Malaysian population. Electrophoresis 2017; 38(17): 2141-9.
[http://dx.doi.org/10.1002/elps.201600471] [PMID: 28524240]

[96]  Srivastava R, Ray S, Vaibhav V, *et al.* Serum profiling of leptospirosis patients to investigate proteomic alterations. J Proteomics 2012; 76(Spec No): 56-68.
[http://dx.doi.org/10.1016/j.jprot.2012.04.007] [PMID: 22554907]

[97]  Mercy CSA, Muthukumaran NS, Velusamy P, *et al.* MicroRNAs regulated by the LPS/TLR2 immune axis as bona fide biomarkers for diagnosis of acute leptospirosis. MSphere 2020; 5(4): e00409-20.
[http://dx.doi.org/10.1128/mSphere.00409-20] [PMID: 32669469]

**CHAPTER 3**

# Phage Therapy as an Alternative Antibacterial Therapy

**Nachimuthu Ramesh[1,*], Prasanth Manohar[2], Archana Loganathan[1], Kandasamy Eniyan[1] and Sebastian Leptihn[2,3,4]**

*[1] Antibiotic Resistance and Phage Therapy Laboratory, School of Bio Sciences and Technology, Vellore Institute of Technology, Vellore, India*

*[2] Zhejiang University-University of Edinburgh (ZJU-UoE) Institute, Zhejiang University, Haining, Zhejiang, P.R.China and The Second Affiliated Hospital Zhejiang University (SAHZU), School of Medicine, Hangzhou, P.R.China*

*[3] Department of Infectious Diseases, Sir Run Run Shaw Hospital, Zhejiang University School of Medicine, Hangzhou, P.R. China*

*[4] Infection Medicine, Biomedical Sciences, Edinburgh Medical School, College of Medicine and Veterinary Medicine, The University of Edinburgh, 1 George Square, Edinburgh, EH8 9JZ, United Kingdom*

**Abstract:** Antibiotic resistance is one of the growing concerns in healthcare settings. Most of the clinical and community (bacterial) strains have grown immune to almost all the available antibiotics. The discovery of new antibiotics or resurging of available antibiotics has failed to outcompete the growing resistance within the bacterial community. Thus, finding an alternative antibacterial modality to treat infectious diseases has become a significant objective among the scientific community around the globe. Phage therapy is one such an antibacterial therapy for the treatment of severe bacterial infections. The bacteriophages (or phage) are viruses that prey on bacteria for their multiplication and survival. Discovery of bacteriophage dates back to the early 1910s when Frederick W. Twort and Felix d'Herelle observed bacteriolytic activity. Before the discovery of antibiotics, phages were the choice of treatment against bacterial infections, but with the inconsistent research, phage therapy lost its importance in the therapeutics. With the emergence of antibiotic resistance, phage therapy and phage research has got a shape to revolutionize the growing bacterial infections. Phage therapy has shown promising results against severe bacterial infections in the circumstances where antibiotic treatment is ineffectual. This emergency has shed light on this forgotten therapy. This chapter will elucidate the history and fundamentals of phage biology and its significance in treating infectious diseases. With the special focus on advancements in phage research and their clinical outcomes which supports the use of phage therapy in humans. It also deals with the

**\* Corresponding Author Nachimuthu Ramesh:** Antibiotic Resistance and Phage Therapy Laboratory, School of Bio Sciences and Technology, Vellore Institute of Technology, Vellore, India; Tel: 9842660673; E-mail: ramesh.n@vit.ac.in

**Parvesh Singh, Vipan Kumar & Rajshekhar Karpoormath (Eds.)**

regulatory inputs required for phage therapy and the commercialization strategies undertaken by pharmaceuticals in the globalization of phage medicine. Besides, the authors would like to brief on the personalized phage therapy and their evolution from lab to bedside endpoints for treating the patients and other future perspectives that hold promise.

**Keywords:** Antibacterials, Antibiotic resistance, Bacteriophages, Bacterial pathogens, *Caudovirales*, Phage resistance, Phage therapy.

## INTRODUCTION

Phage therapy is the use of live bacteriophages (or simply phages) to treat infections caused by pathogenic bacteria. Bacteriophages are known to infect and replicate inside the host bacterium. Bacteriophages are thought to be the widespread, abundant and diverse microorganisms on Earth. The use of bacteriophages for the treatment of bacterial infections can be dated back to 1917; when the bacteriophages were found to kill pathogenic bacteria that were causing diarrhoea and cholera. Though there were improvements in bacteriophage exploration in the 1920s, the discovery of penicillin in 1928 and the subsequent introduction of antibiotics in the 1940s had reduced the applications of bacteriophages in therapy [1]. Antibiotics are antibacterial compounds that are used to kill or inhibit bacteria. Since its introduction as an antibacterial agent, antibiotics have saved millions of lives. As the need for antibiotics started increasing, many pharmaceutical companies were involved in large scale drug discovery from the 1950s to early 1990s. Over half a century antibiotic ruled the medicinal world, until, in the late 1990s the problem of antibiotic resistance has shaken the healthcare sector [2]. Unfortunately, the easy availability of antibiotics paved the way for its misuse and overuse, which eventually leads to resistance among bacteria. As the problem of resistance started increasing, the antibiotic developmental pipeline also becomes dry causing a major crisis to treat bacterial infections. The majority of the infections caused by multi-drug resistant (MDR) bacteria are becoming untreatable and the resistance towards last-resort of antibiotics such as carbapenem, colistin and tigecycline are posing serious threats [3].

Untreatable bacterial infections are causing high mortalities throughout the globe and it was estimated that about 10 million deaths per year by 2050 due to antibiotic-resistant infections [1]. The bacteria that cause hospital-acquired infections (HAI), tuberculosis, co-infections and secondary bacterial infections are becoming difficult to treat. This growing antibiotic crisis is causing a huge burden to the patients both economically and health-related. Though few of the major contributing companies have already stopped their search for new antibiotics, there is still a huge sum of funding available for antibiotics research [4]. The problem with discovering new antibiotics is that there is no guaranty that the bacteria will not develop resistance again. Therefore, there is a need for alternative therapy or non-antibiotic therapy that could be safe, cost-effective, reliable and advantageous. The renewed interest in phage therapy is mainly due to the increasing antibiotic-resistant bacteria and to treat the infections caused by multi-drug resistant bacteria.

## History: From the Vault

The historical evidence for the discovery bacteriophages can be dated back to 1880's, even though the scientific literature explaining these bacteria-eaters are very minimal. Accordingly, in 1896 Hankin reported the antiseptic properties in the water samples collected from Jumna and Ganges Rivers in India [5]. Hankin showed that the antiseptic properties in the water could kill the bacteria, *Vibrio cholerae*. In 1901, Emmerich and Löw described a substance that was causing lysis in the autolysed cultures and it might cure experimental infections but no further experiments were reported [6]. Though there were literature evidences about the reports on bacterial autolysis by Scientists, Gamaleya, Malfitano, Kruse, and Pansini in 1900's, there was no concluding evidence about the action of bacteriophages [7]. Successful improvements in bacteriology, especially bacterial cultures, made significant improvements in bacteriophage research as well, where localized bacteriolysis (plaques) was observed in later years.

The year 2015 marks the century into the 'discovery of bacteriophages' because Frederick W.Twort published his bacteriophage research in 1915 which was considered as the beginning of 'modern phage research'. It was Félix d'Herelle who started working with Twort's phenomenon of 'glassy transformation' and it was later described as bacteriophages. In 1917, d'Herelle described about 'microbes' that were able to lysis the bacteria in the liquid cultures and formed patches on the agar surface, which was termed as 'plaques' [8]. d'Herelle considered them as ultraviruses and later named as 'bacteriophages'. At the Pasteur Institute in Paris, d'Herelle started working with dysentery samples (enteric pathogens) where he identified the lysis of pathogenic bacteria and the formation of clear spots (called as virgin spots) by the invisible microbe. His concept of bacteriophages as the bacterial parasite was found logical. He also hypothesised that bacteriophages require living cells to multiply and interpreted the life cycle as, infection, multiplication, release and reinfection. d'Herelle's research was focused on, (i) the biology of bacteriophages- to understand the biological nature of bacteriophages, and (ii) the therapeutic use of bacteriophages-to cure infectious diseases caused by bacteria. Though the biological nature of bacteriophages was not completely understood, the use of bacteriophages in therapy had overshadowed other biological studies. As soon as d'Herelle observed the increased titres of bacteriophages in the dysentery samples, the concept of phage therapy becomes apparent. The first report of therapeutic use of phages by Bruynoghe and Masin was against staphylococcal infection where the staph phages were injected into the local region of infection [9]. d'Herelle's first attempt to use phages as a prophylactic agent came in 1919 during the outbreak of avian typhosis in France. His reports become more acceptable even at the current standards of research. Later, he investigated phage therapy against bovine haemorrhagic septicaemia. His attempts to prove the safety of phage therapy in humans started with himself being a volunteer (not ethical at current standards), accordingly, after self-administrated phage preparations, he reported no side effects [7]. Later, in the 1920s, the use of phage therapy becomes broad to treat cholera, dysentery, bubonic plaque, conjunctivitis and other skin infections. d'Herelle's standout work was the successful treatment of the cases of bubonic plaque using the antiplaque phages. All the four treated patients recovered rapidly without side effects [10]. In 1920s, there were lots of reports from India about the successful use of phage therapy against cholera [11]. There was lots of enthusiasm to study the bacteriophages and phage therapy in the 1920s but it all came to an end when penicillin was introduced in 1928 by A. Fleming. There were few attempts to prove the efficacy of phage therapy at the clinical stage but the lack of studies to understand the nature of bacteriophages had substantial concern and negative impact. In the subsequent years, the success and the availability of antibiotics had ceased the phage therapy clinical trials in the United States and in most of the European countries. But, the Soviet Union and other Eastern European countries continued their research on phage therapy, especially, at the Eliava Institute.

In the post-antibiotic era (after 2000), in which, the bacteria are resisting the antibacterial effects of antibiotics; there is a renewed interest to study and to use bacteriophages as an alternative. Despite of the halted clinical applications of bacteriophages, the basic research on phage biology kept-going and some of the major discoveries were made (Fig. **1**); (a) in 1934- phage therapy clinical trials were performed with the lack of controls, low efficacy and using impure phage lysates, (b) in 1939- Ellis and Delbrück demonstrated the phage life cycle as adsorption, growth within the host and lysis, (c) in 1940- Ruska provided the first electron microscopic images of bacteriophage, (d) in 1982- Sanger published the first phage genome report of lambda bacteriophage, (e) in 1985- phage therapy was used to treat infections such as septicaemia and meningitis caused by multi-drug resistant bacteria, (f) in 1992- the efficacy of phage therapy was studied using animal models (Soothill *et al.*), (g) in 2006- the introduction of phage-based biocontrol agents against *L. monocytogenes*, (h) in 2009- controlled phase I/II clinical trials to treat MDR *P. aeruginosa* (Wright *et al.*) [12], (i) in 2015- multicentre phase I/II trials against burn wound patients (Phagoburn) [13], (j) in

2017- successful treatment of *A. baumannii* infections (Schooley *et al.*) [14], (k) in 2019- engineered bacteriophages were used to treat drug-resistant *M. abscessus* infections (Dedrick *et al.*) [15]. The research on bacteriophage biology and phage therapy started growing at the rapid phase after 2015, and they are considered as one of the best alternatives to cure multi-drug resistant bacterial infections.

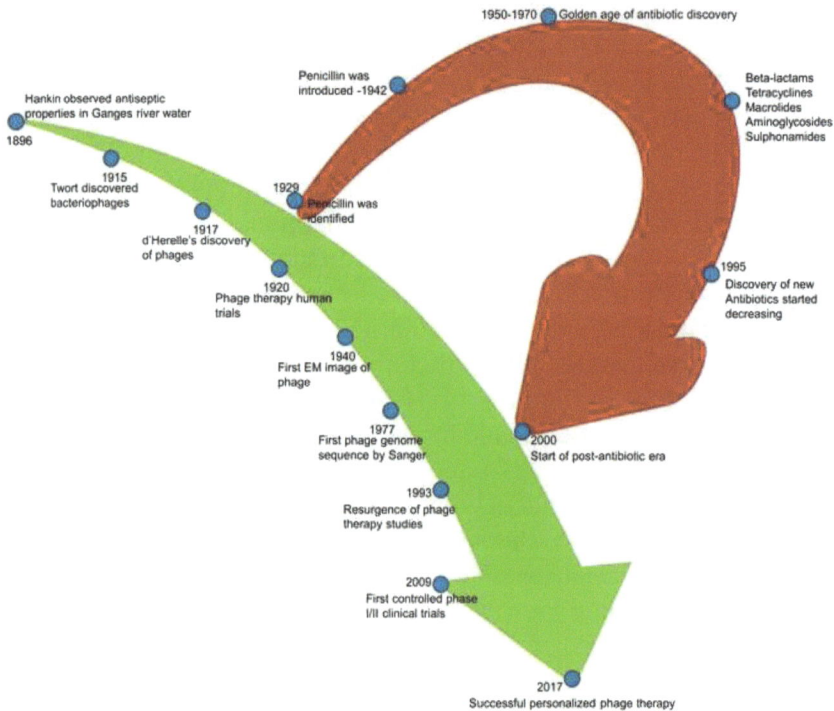

**Fig. (1).** History of bacteriophage discovery and the evolution of phage therapy through the years. (Green-bacteriophage discovery, red-antibiotics discovery).

## Basics: Phage Life cycle and Phage Biology

The bacteriophage life cycle can be differentiated into various stages such as, 1) attachment of bacteriophages on to the bacterial host, 2) injection of phage genetic material into the host, 3) synthesis of new phage proteins inside the host using the bacterial machinery, 4) lysis of host bacterium and the release of new phage progeny particles (Fig. **2**) [16]. During the infection process, phages bind to the specific receptors on the bacterial cell surface and inject the genetic material. After the injection of genetic material, phage follows one of the two cycles, lytic (virulent) and lysogenic (temperate). Lytic phages immediately take over the bacterial cell machinery to produce phage components. Then they assemble inside the host bacterium and lyse (destroy) the bacterium to release new phage particles.

In the case of lysogenic phages, the genetic material of the phage is incorporated into the host chromosome and replicate with it, without destroying the host bacterium. Under certain conditions, lysogenic phages start producing phage proteins and destroy the bacterium to release new phage particles. When induced, some of the lysogenic phages can follow lytic cycle. For phage therapy, lytic phages are preferred, especially, to destroy or kill the target bacteria immediately after infection. The lytic phages used for therapy should not undergo lysogenic cycle at any conditions because the incorporation of phage genetic material into the pathogenic bacterium might lead to other serious complications, which require another therapy for treatment [17].

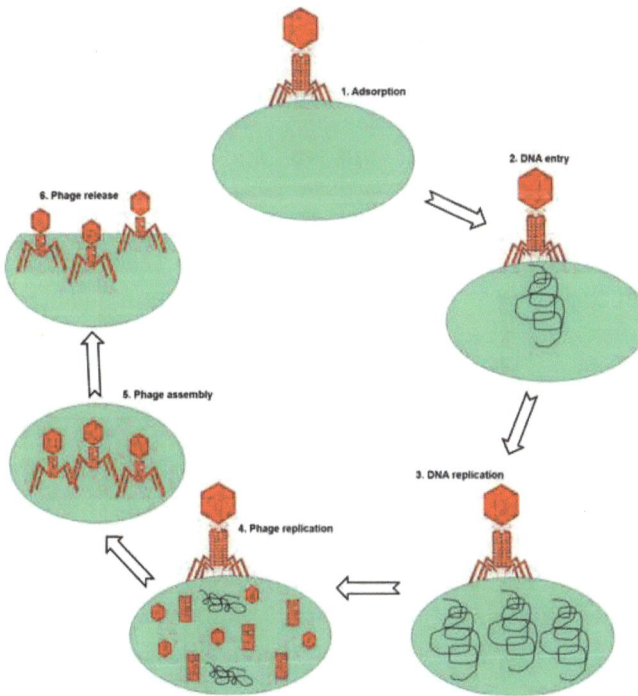

**Fig. (2).** Life cycle of lytic phages. **1)** Bacteriophages adsorb to the bacterial cell, **2)** Phages inject the genetic material inside the bacterium, **3)** Replication of phage DNA inside the bacteria, **4)** Production of phage structures, **5)** Assembly of phage particles, **6)** Bacterial lysis and release of phage particles.

Most of the phages are infectious to their bacterial host only when they carry their complementary receptor, usually receptors are present in the outer membrane of the bacteria. The specificity of lytic phages will be altered based on their receptors and the determination of phage host range is upon their receptor binding ability. Usually, phages are said to be host specific but that is not always true because nowadays phages with broad-host ranges were identified, which are infecting more than one strain or species or even genus of bacteria [18]. On the other hand, phage-resistant mechanisms in the bacteria have evolved through years that eventually make the phages to evolve equally to break the resistance barrier. The well-known resistance mechanisms in bacteria includes alteration of phage-binding receptors and CRISPR/Cas systems (Clustered Regularly Interspaced Palindromic Repeats/CRISPR-associated system), while for phages, recognition of alternative binding receptors and anti-CRISPR proteins were identified [19 - 21]. The phage-resistance mechanisms are discussed in detail under the sub-heading 'phage resistant bacterial evolution'. The lytic phages that are associated with human pathogens and gut microbiota are included in the orders *Caudovirales* (dsDNA, tailed phages) and *Microviridae* (ssDNA, tailless) which will be discussed in the following section.

**Taxonomical Classification of Bacteriophages**

The taxonomical classification of viruses and their subsequent naming is maintained by "International Committee on Taxonomy of Viruses" (ICTV). The classification of bacteriophage is maintained by another ICTV sub-committee called "Bacterial and Archaeal Subcommittee" (BAVS). The bacteriophages are classified based on their genome (DNA/RNA; ss/ds), morphology, enveloped or not, their host-range, and genomic sequence similarities [22 - 24]. The tailed phages or dsDNA phages are classified under the order *Caudovirales*. The classification in 1999 was based on the phage morphology which had three families, (I) *Myoviridae* - long contractile tails, (II) *Siphoviridae* – long non-contractile tails, (III) *Podoviridae* – short non-contractile tails. *Siphoviridae* are known to be the most abundant tailed phages. With the advancements in the Next Generation Sequencing (NGS) techniques, the genomic and metagenomic projects on phages have increased. Though the earlier classification had not included genome diversity, the availability of genome comparison tools has made phage classification possible at the genome level. Later in 2018, the ICTV grouped all the tailed phages into five families, 1) *Ackermannviridae*, 2) *Herelleviridae*, 3) *Myoviridae*, 4) *Podoviridae* and 5) *Siphoviridae* [25]. Both *Ackermannviridae* and *Herelleviridae* are morphologically similar to *Myoviridae*.

The extended ICTV classification of *Caudovirales* (tailed, dsDNA phages) was updated recently in 2019 (Fig. **3**) (https://talk.ictvonline.org/taxonomy/) that included 9 families, 44 subfamilies, 671 genera and 1967 species, and the genus *Lilyvirus* has one species. Up to date, a total of 2914 complete genome sequences of bacteriophages of the order *Caudovirales* are deposited in public databases (https://www.ncbi.nlm.nih.gov/genomes/GenomesGroup.cgi?taxid=28883#).

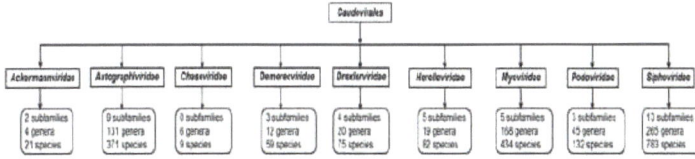

**Fig. (3).** Classification of *Caudovirales* bacteriophages based on the new (2019) ICTV classification.

## Family: *Ackermannviridae*

The family *Ackermannviridae* contains two subfamilies, *Aglimvirinae* and *Cvivirinae*, with a total of 4 genera with 21 species. At present, 23 complete genome sequences are available within this family. The common host species includes *Salmonella, Shigella, Dickeya, Escherichia, Klebsiella, Serratia* and *Erwinia* phages (Fig. **4**).

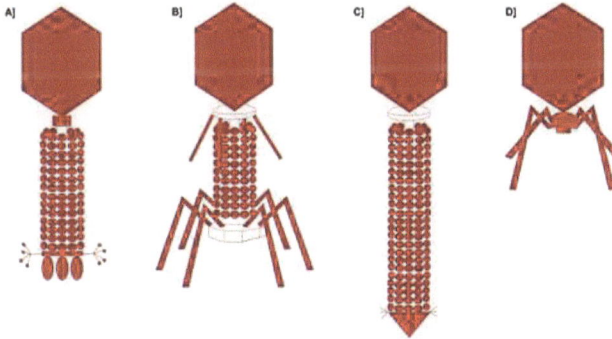

**Fig. (4).** Morphological classification of *Caudovirales* bacteriophages, **A)** *Ackermannviridae*, **B)** *Myoviridae* and *Chaseviridae* and *Herelleviridae*, **C)** *Siphoviridae* and *Demerecviridae* and *Drexlerviridae*, **D)** *Podoviridae* and *Autographiviridae*. Genome diversity can be observed within these families.

## Family: *Autographiviridae*

Though this taxonomic classification was proposed in 2008, the new analysis included 9 subfamilies (*Beijerinckvirinae, Colwellvirinae, Corkvirinae, Krylovirinae, Melnykvirinae, Molineuxvirinae, Okabevirinae, Slopekvirinae* and *Studiervirinae*) with 131 genera, 371 species. There are 362 complete genome sequences available. The classification of this sub-family was based on the presence of single-subunit RNA polymerase (>100 kDa) with most of the virus possessing a small head and a short tail similar to *Podoviridae* (Fig. **4**). The common phages within this family include *Acinetobacter, Vibrio, Marinomonas, Pseudomonas, Pectobacterium, Dickeya, Yersinia, Cronobacter, Salmonella* sp. Based on the shared homologous/orthologous proteins, the genomic relations were redefined, and the *Autographiviridae* family was proposed for classification in 2008 by Lavigne *et al.* [26].

## Family: *Chaseviridae*

This family was named as a tribute to Martha Cowles Chase, with the first phage isolated was φEcoM-GJ1 [27]. Most of the phages in this family belong to *Myoviridae,* having isometric head and contractile tails, with hosts belonging to the Gammaproteobacteria class. It contains six genera and nine species but no subfamilies; a total of 8 whole genome sequences are available.

## Family: *Demerecviridae*

This new family contains 3 subfamilies (*Ermolyevavirinae, Markadamsvirinae,* and *Mccorquodalevirinae*), 12 genera, 59 species encompassing 58 whole genome sequences. The common hosts are *Aeromonas, Escherichia, Klebsiella, Pectobacterium, Proteus, Providencia, Salmonella, Shigella, Vibrio,* and *Yersinia* species. The nomenclature of this family is credited to Milislav Demerec for his works on bacteriophage; he was one of the pioneers to isolate *E. coli* phage T5 in 1945 [28].

## Family: *Drexlerviridae*

*Drexlerviridae* is glorified for Henry Drexler, who worked with T1-like phages. This group of bacteriophages had found numerous name changes such as *T1-likevirus* to *Tunavirus.* The present classification contains 4 subfamilies (*Braunvirinae, Rogunavirinae, Tempevirinae,* and *Tunavirinae*), 20 genera and 75 species with 71 annotated whole genomes available. A series of taxonomic changes have been amended to this family, and the host is dominated by *Escherichia,* but other strains such as *Cronobacter, Enterobacter, Klebsiella, Pantoea,* and *Shigella*-specific isolates are also seen.

## Family: *Herelleviridae*

This family has been named after Félix d'Hérelle in remembrance of the 100th anniversary of the discovery of bacteriophages. A large portion of the viruses in this family is of myovirus with the hosts belonging to *Firmicutes* phylum. The phages are classified by features such as terminase large subunit, major capsid protein, tail tube, tail sheath, and tail tape measure protein. *Herelleviridae* consists of 5 subfamilies (*Bastillevirinae, Brockvirinae, Jasinkavirinae, Spounavirinae,* and *Twortvirinae*), 19 genera, 82 species, and 120 complete genomes are currently available.

## Family: *Myoviridae*

These are some of the most common therapeutic phage families containing long contractile tail with sheath and central tube (Fig. **4**). In the 8th ICTV report [29], the *Myoviridae* comprised of 5 genera of bacteriophages while the recently updated list comprised of 5 subfamilies (*Eucampyvirinae, Ounavirinae, Peduovirinae, Tevenvirinae,* and *Vequintavirinae*), 168 genera, 434 species with 624 whole genome sequences. A separate family was proposed and introduced to *Caudovirales* in 2017 [30].

**Family: *Podoviridae***

They are a family of short-tailed phages (Fig. **4**) containing three subfamilies (*Picovirinae, Rakietenvirinae,* and *Sepvirinae*), 45 genera, and 132 species comprising of 239 complete genome sequences available. This includes phages such as *T7-like*, the *P22-like*, *429-like*, and the *N4-like* phages while their genome contains inverted terminal repeats [26].

**Family: *Siphoviridae***

These are one of the largest family comprises of 13 subfamilies (*Arquatrovirinae, Bclasvirinae, Chebruvirinae, Dclasvirinae, Dolichocephalovirinae, Guernsey-virinae, Langleyhallvirinae, Mccleskeyvirinae, Mclasvirinae, Nclasvirinae, Nymbaxtervirinae, Pclasvirinae,* and *Tybeckvirinae*), 265 genera, 783 species, and 1407 complete genome sequences. These phages are made up of long non-contractile tails with an icosahedral protein head (Fig. **4**).

**Genus: *Lilyvirus***

As of now, *Lilyvirus* contains one species and one genome sequence is available that belong to *Paenibacillus* sp. Based on the NCBI complete genome sequences list, there are two unclassified *Caudovirales* genomes that are not classified under any families.

**Key Advantages and Disadvantages of Phage Therapy**

Phage therapy is considered as one of the efficient therapies to overcome the problem of antibiotic-resistance, and there are considerable advantages and under-studied disadvantages to be discussed.

Some of the advantages of using phage therapy are [17, 31, 32], 1. Easy availability- bacteriophages can be found everywhere with their bacterial niche, therefore, easily discoverable; 2. Host specificity- bacteriophages are usually specific to their host bacterium, which means they do not disturb the normal flora during the treatment; 3. Self-replicating- bacteriophages can multiply in the presence of the host bacterium, therefore, during therapy a single dose of phages is sufficient to reduce the bacterial load (auto-dosing); 4. Lytic bacteriophages are natural bactericidal agents; 5. No toxicity- bacteriophages are made of proteins and nucleic acids, therefore, no inherent toxicity; 6. Formulation- bacteriophages can be readily combined with antibiotics or any other antibacterial agents for treat benefits; 7. Biofilm clearance- bacteriophages can produce depolymerases that can degrade bacterial exopolymers to kill biofilm cells; 8. Low cost- phage therapy is expected to be available at lesser cost than antibiotics because with modern technologies phage production (purification) costs can be relatively low.

There are some disadvantages in using phage therapy [17, 31] and we have discussed the solutions to overcome the disadvantages in Table **1**.

**Table 1. Phage therapy: Notable disadvantages and their remedies.**

| S. No. | Disadvantages | How to Overcome? |
|---|---|---|
| 1. | **Selection of phages**- not all the phages can be used for therapy, only lytic phages should be selected. Using lysogenic phages can lead to other therapeutic complications. | Screening for lytic phages at the initial phage isolation process will eliminate the problem. |
| 2. | **Narrow host range**- phages have minimal target range to infect specific strain or species or genus of bacteria. | Using phage cocktails (combination of phages) will make the target broader; in addition, phages are known to have synergy with antibiotics. |
| 3. | **Immune response**- As a pharmaceutical agent, bacteriophage is protein-based, live microorganism that can induce immune responses but the level of responses are not well-studied. | There are protein-based drugs that are already in use against many diseases. No adverse side effects have been reported from the countries that are already using phages for treatment. |
| 4. | **Unusual drug**- phages are bacterial viruses, therefore, using viruses in therapy needs public awareness. There are lack of proper clinical guidelines, regulatory guidelines and cGMP guidelines for phage production and treatment. | There are studies that are focussed on phage therapy clinical trials and a proper regulatory framework has to be designed to overcome these major hurdles. |

## PHAGE THERAPY: PHAGE RESISTANT BACTERIAL EVOLUTION

Bacteria-phage co-evolution is important for the ecological and evolutionary processes within microbial communities. Though the development of phage resistance in the bacteria is a natural process, the impact of such a resistance during phage therapy is one of the important concerns. Accordingly, there are some of the important mechanisms of phage resistance in the bacteria;
**1)** Preventing phage adsorption: Adsorption of phages to the bacterial cell is one of the initial steps in phage infection, therefore, bacteria develop different adsorption blocking mechanisms including: a) blocking of phage receptors on the bacterial outer membrane [19, 33], b) the production of extracellular matrix (polymers) to prevent phages from attaching to their receptors [19, 34], and c) the

production of inhibitors to block the phage receptors (making a competitive environment) [19, 35]. **2)** Entry of phage DNA is prevented using the superinfection exclusion (Sie) proteins that block the entry of phage DNA into the bacterium causing immunity against phages [36, 37]. Sie systems are well-studied in both Gram-positive and Gram-negative bacteria [37, 38]. **3)** Cutting phage nucleic acids: a) Restriction-modification (R-M) systems are almost found in all the bacteria, which mainly protect the cell from invading (viral) DNA [39 - 42], b) The CRISPR-Cas systems are one of the recently identified mechanisms that are involved in phage multiplication [43, 44], c) Defence islands: Genes that are involved in bacterial defence systems are clustered in specific genome loci. It is known as 'DISARM system' that is associated with bacterial innate defence and functions similar to R-M systems [45, 46]. **4)** Abortive infection (Abi) systems provide resistance through the abortion of phage infection. Rex system found in *E. coli* strains is one of the best studied Abi systems [19, 47]. There are other newly discovered defence systems in bacteria that include Thoeris systems (ThsAB) in *Bacillus* that targets *Myoviridae* phages, Hachiman systems against *Bacillus* phages and Zorya (type I and type II) and Druantia (DruE) [48].

The occurrence of phage-resistant bacteria is a natural process, the same can happen during therapy, in which, the pathogenic bacteria can resist phage infection that can result in treatment failure. But the appearance of phage-resistant bacteria is not uncommon during therapy. The previous reports of phage-resistance found in after treatment were, Smith and Huggins observed the presence of phage-resistant bacterial strains in *E. coli* while treating mouse meningitis model using phage R [49], in another study Smith *et al.* reported the phage-resistant *E. coli* strains in calf diarrhoea model [50] and the presence of phage-resistance was observed against *S. aureus* after treating a 16-year old boy for 3 months using phages (but the problem was overcame by using different phage preparations) [51]. The recorded experimental data showed that phage-resistant bacterial variants were noted in 80% and 50% of the studies that included intestinal and sepsis models [52]. Few clinical trials also reported the emergence of phage resistance after treatment [52]. But the development of phage-resistance is not without causing the fitness-cost in bacteria. The phage-resistant bacterial variants were analysed and showed that the mutations or mechanisms that confer resistance result in the loss of important bacterial characteristics such as virulence [53]. Though the phage therapy treatment centres haven't reported any treatment failure due to phage resistant bacterial pathogens, the appearance of phage resistance should not be underestimated and needs further investigation. The use of phage cocktails and phage-antibiotic combinations are well-studied alternatives at the laboratory level, and personalized phage therapy is another therapeutic alternative to tackle the emergence of phage resistance.

## Phage Cocktails and Personalized Phage Therapy

The use of phage cocktails is one of the important therapeutic alternatives to avoid the development of phage-resistance during treatment (Table **2**). By combining multiple phages it is possible to broaden the phage infectivity and increase the number of target pathogens. The phages present in the phage cocktail act in synergism to attack multiple targets (receptors) in the bacteria that eventually reduces the development of bacterial co-resistance (Fig. **5**) [54]. Gu *et al.* reported the importance of using phage cocktails in reducing the emergence of phage-resistant *K. pneumoniae* mutants [55]. Studies also reported that when phage cocktails were used the emergence of phage resistance was delayed or decreased against *E. coli* [56, 57]. This approach is also used by Georgian phage therapy centres to treat patients, notably for empirical treatments, but the phage combinations tend to change at the regular basis to adapt to the most prevalent pathogens [58, 59]. The personalized phage therapy uses a single phage or phage cocktails against the pathogen/s isolated from the patient and the phage formulations are prepared from the phage bank [59]. In one of the phage therapy clinical trials that used monotherapy (single phage) to treat infected patients showed that there were some modifications in the pathogens (identified using phage typing) after phage treatment which might escape the phage infection [60, 61]. A case report by Schooley *et al.* showed the successful treatment of a patient infected with MDR *A. baumannii* using personalized phage therapy [62]. Another study reported the use of personalized phage therapy to treat lung transplant patient infected with MDR *P. aeruginosa* and during the treatment phage susceptibility was monitored throughout and the new phages were used as soon as phage resistance was emerged [63]. The occurrence of phage resistance was not immediate; they were noted after continuous treatment for more than a month. In another study, the combination of six bacteriophages was used to treat *P. aeruginosa* urinary tract infection and the results showed that the bacterial count was reduced sharply after phage treatment and there was no appearance of phage resistance during or after the therapy [64]. A recent study also suggests that phage resistance can be avoided if the bacterial exposure to the phages is in mixtures or combinations, where the order of phage exposure determines the fitness cost in bacteria [53]. Therefore, it should be noted that phage resistance is not prohibitive to phage therapy but the emergence of resistant strains should be carefully monitored and immediate alternative phage composition should be used for treatment.

**Table 2. Recent studies investigating the efficacy of phage cocktails in treatment.**

| Target Bacteria | Model | Phage Cocktail and Dosing | Comments | References |
|---|---|---|---|---|
| *Escherichia coli* | Murine bacteremia | 3 phages and 1 × $10^6$ PFU/mouse | Fewer phage resistant bacteria appeared in cocktail | [65] |
| *Klebsiella pneumoniae* | Burn wound infections in mice | 5 phages encapsulated in liposome and $10^8$ PFU/ml | Liposomal phage cocktails saved all the animals | [66] |
| *Klebsiella pneumoniae* | Burn wound infections in mice | 5 phages and $10^8$ PFU/ml | Phage cocktail gave maximum protection compared to single phage | [67] |
| *Pseudomonas aeruginosa* | Burn wound infections in randomized trial | 12 phages and 1 × $10^6$ PFU/ml | Effective at low concentrations but at slow rate | [13] |
| MDR *Acinetobacter baumannii* | Treatment of 68-year-old diabetic patient | 9 phages and $\approx 10^9$ PFU/dose | Patient recovered from the infection | [14] |
| MDR *Mycobacterium abscessus* subsp. *massiliense* | Treatment of 15-year-old cystic fibrosis patient | 3 phages and $10^9$ PFU/dose of each phage | First therapeutic use of phages for human mycobacteria infections with clinical improvements | [15] |
| *Pseudomonas aeruginosa* | Acute respiratory infections in mice | 2 phages and MOI of 0.05 | Reducing the respiratory bacterial burden in 48h | [68] |
| *Pseudomonas aeruginosa* | Bacteremia in *Galleria mellonella* | 2 phages and MOI of 8 & 25 | Larval survival rate increases with dose | [69] |
| Multiple bacteria- *E. coli*, *K. pneumoniae* and *E. cloacae* | Bacteremia in *Galleria mellonella* | 3 phages and $10^4$ PFU/ml | 100% larval survival rate was obtained with five doses at 6h interval | [69] |
| Methicillin-resistant *Staphylococcus aureus* (MRSA) | Soft tissue infections in rats | 2 phages and encapsulated phage cocktails | The transfersome-entrapped phage cocktails saved all the infected animals | [70] |
| *Staphylococcus aureus* | Peri-prosthetic joint infections in rats | 5 phages and $10^9$ PFU/ml | Decreased inflammation within joints when treated with phage and vancomycin | [71] |
| *Staphylococcus aureus* | Mastitis in mice | 2 phages and $10^9$ PFU/ml | The highest intramammary phage titer was achieved without spreading systematically | [72] |

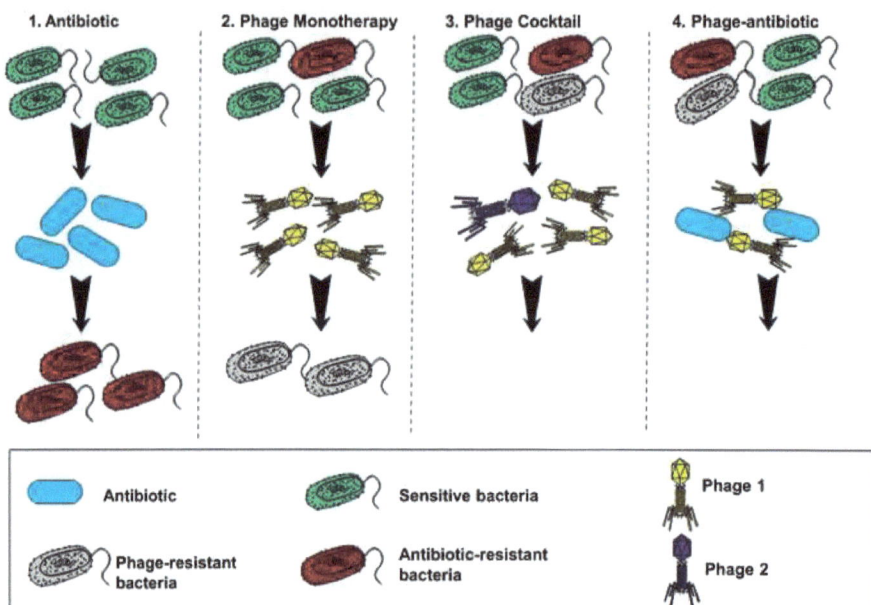

**Fig. (5).** Strategies to tackle the development of antibiotic resistance and phage resistance. **1)** antibiotic resistant bacteria emerges during antibiotic therapy, **2)** occurrence of phage resistance during phage monotherapy, **3)** elimination of phage resistance using phage cocktails (use of more than one phage), **4)** combination of phage and antibiotics to kill the pathogenic bacteria.

## Phage-Antibiotics Synergy

Bacteria can resist antibiotics using the several known mechanisms such as decreased expression of targets, increased drug efflux or decreased drug in-take, major changes in metabolic pathways, *etc.* Few of the well characterized phage resistant mechanisms are discussed earlier. On the other hand, the combination of phage-antibiotics can act in synergism to fight against bacteria that eventually increases the therapeutic efficacy [73]. The combination of ciprofloxacin and phages was found to inhibit the emergence of phage-resistant mutants during *K. pneumoniae* treatment [74]. In another study, *S. aureus* was treated with gentamicin and phages to prevent the emergence of phage resistance [75]. The potential benefit of combining phages and streptomycin was noted against *P. aeruginosa* [76]. The phage-antibiotic synergism was also observed against *B. cepacia* and *P. aeruginosa* [77, 78]. In addition, the phages (in the phage-antibiotic combination) that are targeting the bacterial receptors that are part of the antibiotic resistance mechanisms such as efflux pumps can restore antibiotic susceptibility [79]. The selective pressure caused by phages can alter the resistance pattern in bacteria making it re-sensitize to antibiotics [80]. Many studies proved the phage-antibiotic synergism against Gram-positive and Gram-negative bacteria [81]. It was also noted that the stress caused by beta-lactam antibiotics makes the cells more filamentous or swelled leading to increased phage production. The adsorption efficacy of phages did not change with the enlarged bacterial cells [81]. In addition, the anti-biofilm activity of phage-antibiotic was studied that showed synergistic effect against biofilm-forming bacteria such as *S. aureus* and *P. aeruginosa* [82 - 84]. Therefore, the combination of phage-antibiotic can reduce the development of phage resistance as well as improve the therapeutic efficacy.

## IMMUNOLOGICAL ASPECTS OF PHAGE THERAPY

Phage-human interaction is an interrelationship between bacteriophages that circulate within the human body and the mammalian cells [85]. The role of phage and human cell interaction has become very important criteria to determine the clinical outcome and the effect of phage therapy on the human system [86]. Thus, phage-human interplay has become a crucial part of therapy to be explored by the researchers for designing effective phage therapeutics. In recent years, there are many studies which showed the interaction of phages, bacteria, and the mammalian immune system. Despite few disadvantages being reported, yet many studies have come up with significant advantages in phage-immune system interaction in evading bacterial infections. This outcome has opened a broad field of research in phage therapy which includes phage evolution in humans during therapy and the immune responses during phage therapy.

### Phage Transverse and Human Phageome

Phages are ubiquitous [87] and the natural phageome population in the human body is highly diversified [88]. The presence of phages in the human body is right from birth till death and found to be the most abundant biological entities in the human body. The virome population is found to outnumber other microbial populations, and they are highly complex in the intestinal environment [89]. Bacteriophages are the fundamental viruses in the gastro-intestine and it was estimated to have about ten trillion phages in the intestinal cavity [90]. Phages are found in blood, lymph, spinal fluid, and other organs (fluids) that were believed to be sterile previously.

Apart from phageome, injected therapeutic phages are still considered to be the foreign bodies by the immune system and thus, produce an immune response. These immune responses are caused by the release of endotoxins as the phage kill the bacterial host by multiplication [91, 92]. Phages are found to be highly populated in the gut region of the human body. The gut region is estimated to carry approximately $5.09 \times 10^{10}$ Plaque Forming Units per gram of the faeces [90, 93]. The continuous stream of phages is found to be disseminated from the gut and reaches the other parts of the body. But how these bacteriophages are transversed across the various organs of the human body remains a mystery for researchers. Few fundamental studies on the phage distribution and translocation have unlocked the future of phage biology and have laid a path to improve phage therapy outcome. Phages use different strategies to travel and explore the human system. The rapid translocation of phages from the parental route to other organs remains not fully understood but one reason might be due to the bacterial invasion. Few studies have hypothesized the transfer mechanisms that includes transcytosis, translocation through damaged barriers ("leaky guts" as described in the literature), and by hiding inside the mammalian epithelial cells ("Trojan Horse" as described in the literature) (Fig. **6**). These translocation mechanisms help in the distribution and establishment of phage population across the human system [94].

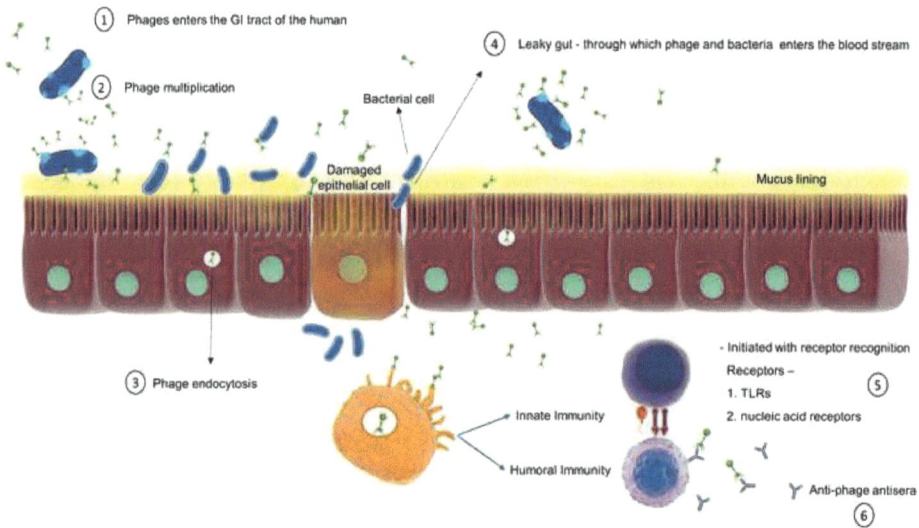

**Fig. (6).** Immune responses produced in the GI (Gastrointestinal) tract in response to the bacteriophages. **1)** Entry of phage into the GI tract, **2)** Phages multiply on finding a suitable host, **3)** Phage endocytosis by the epithelial cells, **4)** Damaged epithelial cells causing leaky guts, through which phages and bacteria enters the blood, **5)** Phages encountered by the macrophages initiate innate immune responses by recognizing the receptors, **6)** Humoral immune response against the phage by producing anti-phage antisera (created with somersault1824.com and BioRender.com).

Transcytosis is best described in the study conducted by Nguger *et al.*, 2018, in which the T4 phage transcytosis through epithelial cells was examined [95]. The microscopic analysis of confluent epithelial cells showed the occurrence of natural phages in the human body even in the absence of bacterial infections and this circulation is found to be supported through the transcytosis mechanism [96].

Translocation through damaged barriers or leaky guts is a random mechanism of phage itself because this depends on the damages in the epithelial cells or might need a special adaption in the gene function to break the barrier; such evidence was highlighted in the streptococcal phage. The streptococcal phages have adapted the ability to produce hyaluronidase that degrades the connective tissues, thereby, facilitating the translocation of phages [19, 97]. The Trojan horse mechanism of translocation is mediated by the receptor recognized endocytosis by the action of epithelial cells.

The mucous lining of the gut aids in preventing the translocation of phages into the bloodstream and the surrounding tissues, thereby, acting as the first line of defence for producing an immune response by the phage proteins. Phages concentrate in the mucus by a weak interaction mediated by Ig-like folds in phage structural proteins [98]. A study conducted by Nguyen *et al.*, 2017 revealed that phages are transposed through the endomembrane system of Golgi bodies. This study also found that 31 billion phages are translocated per day from the human gut system [95]. The transportation of bacteriophages in the epithelial cells is bidirectional, which can pass through vesicular as well the cytosolic compartments from apical to the basal direction. This was confirmed by using *in vivo* studies in which the transcytosis was analysed microscopically using the gut, lung, liver and brain cell lines [95, 99].

## Phage-Immune System Crosstalk

The immune system is stimulated by the responses when the foreign particle (called as antigen) enters the human body. During phage therapy the immune responses can happen upon infection. The major components that are released during the phage infection are the bacterial cell debris and the endotoxins. The humoral immune system has a very strong response against the foreign molecule that enters the human body. This type of immune function is mediated by the production of antibodies. Humoral immunity plays a vital role during the phage treatment, as they are mainly involved in defending against extracellular microbes and endotoxins [100]. In most of the clinical cases, there was an immune reaction observed when phage is administered to the patient. This intertwined response of the human body is a result of the release of bacteria-associated molecules released during the bacterial killing. Despite this, studies showed the importance of inducing the immune reaction during phage therapy. The clinical evidences available for the immunological changes that results during phage therapy is a less studied topic in phage biology [101].

Information concerning the anti-phage humoral reaction during phage treatment is still very scant. Each phage has a specific and unique marker that induces a specific immune response in an individual. The immune response or anti-phage antibody produced is directly proportional to the different variants of phages that circulates in the system [102]. Thus, showing increased anti-phage antibodies during phage cocktail administration than in single phage treatment. The human immune system remains to be one of the complex systems to understand. Induction of multi-variant anti-phage antibodies during the phage cocktail administration has become a great hurdle to relate the interlace between immune response and the outcome of phage treatment, therefore, many immunological responses remains undiscovered [103]. Intestine helps in maintaining the body homeostasis. The epithelial cells are actively involved in antigen processing and immune cell regulations. Phages are found in the infants (new born) transferred vertically through placenta (mother to infant) [103]. This is known to keep the immune system active from the birth. A study by Gorski *et al.*, 2005 showed that the endogenous virome population in the intestinal system helps the human body to maintain the immunological homeostasis by producing the immune modules [104].

The studies on the efficacy of phage therapy in the immunosuppressed patients have shown that these patients tend to show a little effect when phages (alone) are used to treat bacterial infections. Adjacent to this, the phage populating in an individual has shown to reflect the health status of an individual. It was further suggested that virulent or lytic phage aids in the diversification and ecological evolution of the microbiome in an individual. This was supported by the evidences shown in one of the studies, in which, the phageome of immunodeficient patients were found to be quiet less compared to the immunologically active individuals [105]. The reports on the pre-clinical studies of phage therapy in immunocompromised patients are not explored to date. The other aspects of the phages as the immunosuppressive drug needed to be assessed. The disadvantages of phages in the immunosuppressed or immunodeficient patients may create a random or altered immune response, which might increase the chances of mortality in patients. A study conducted on phage therapy in allergic disorder patients showed that allergic reaction was observed on 1.4% of the patients subjected to phage therapy. Few studies have also shown that phage therapy in allergic patients had no negative reaction, such as in phi X174 phage administered intravenously in patient with hyper-IgE syndrome [106, 107].

## Bacteriophage and Innate Immune Response

The innate immune response for endogenous phages or during the phage therapy is initiated by recognizing the phage genome (DNA and RNA). This frontline defence mechanism comprises of phagocytic cells that are involved in phage endocytosis [108]. The family of innate immune system senses the pathogens

through a set of receptors such as nucleic acid receptors and Toll-like receptors (TLRs). These receptors sense the pathogen recognition receptors (PRR) on the bacteriophages stimulating an inflammatory response. Phage processing by the innate immune response involves the series of steps and they can be divided as,
1) Phagocytic cell recognition,
2) Endocytic recognition and processing, and
3) Cytoplasmic recognition and processing. Phagocytic cell recognition and endocytic recognition is mediated by the interaction between PRR and the sensors in phagocytic cells, while the cytoplasmic recognition and processing are mediated by Retinoic acid-inducible gene I (RIG-1)-like receptors and cyclic-di-nucleotide (CDN). The process of phage recognition begins with engulfing the circulating phages, after which the exposure of the PRR and the receptors on the phagocytic cells sense the exposed PRR. Pathogen recognition receptors on the bacteriophages are sensed by the number of TLRs (1, 2, 4, 5, 6, and 11), for example, the TLR3 binds dsRNA of the phage nucleic acid. Cytoplasmic recognition is developed in intracellular bacteriophages, they are initiated upon release of phage DNA in the cytoplasm by phage induced bacterial lysis [109].

## Bacteriophage and Humoral Immune Response

The effect of translocated phage and the humoral immune response is one of the unexplored fields of phage research. The generation of neutralizing antibodies to the phages have been demonstrated in some of the earlier studies [102]. Studies by Kucharewicz-Krukowska and Bruttin have shown that the anti-phage antibodies are induced when phage is administered locally, and there was less evidence of anti-phage antibodies produced during oral administration, which enlightened that humoral immune response depends on the route of phage administration [110, 111]. The phage inactivation during therapy can lead to the loss of phage viability, thus reducing their efficacy. Few studies have reported the inactivation of phages on binding to the neutralizing antibodies. Dabrowska *et al.*, 2014 found that antibodies sensitized against T4 phage were highly specific to the protein coat, which decreased the activity of phages by changing their physical nature [112]. The inactivation of phages can take place due to external factors such as phage aggregation, binding of phage to dead cells, *etc.* The effect of phage inactivation by the production of neutralizing anti-phage antibodies assessed by Dabrowska *et al.*, 2014 showed that phage aggregation or destabilization of phage capsid was the major reason for the loss of phage viability [112]. When formulating phage therapy, the dosage has to be taken into consideration as 20% of the phages are cleared by the neutralizing antibodies and phagocytosis [86, 113].

The rate of neutralizing antibodies produced is directly proportional to the number of binding bacteriophages and other external factors. Most of the studies have shown the varying ability of phage binding and anti-phage production in response to phage sensitization in both *in vitro* and *In vivo* methods. The phage formulation largely depends on the bacteria that are colonizing the site of infection in the patients, based on the above criteria, the phage can either be administered as single or in cocktails [114]. Homogenous phage administration has shown productive immune response than the heterogenous phage challenge. Immune response studies against the heterogenous phage population are tedious because phages have a unique receptors that are recognized by the variant of antibodies [115]. Thus, enumerating the anti-phage antibodies against the relative phages added the disadvantage to the experimental outcomes. Any notable immune response against the phages brings a question on the efficacy of phage therapy in the long run. Understanding the phage-immune cell interrelationship could bring an effective strategy for the treatment of clinical infections.

**Synergistic Interaction of the Human Immune System and Phages**

Even though there is great evidence for the loss of phage viability to antibodies during phage therapy as well as for the endogenous phages, their presence is sometimes regarded as an advantage by the researchers [116]. The study conducted by Zaczek *et al.*, 2016 showed that the MS-1 phage cocktail given orally or locally in 20 patients produced the anti-phage antibody responses, but those responses didn't alter or affect the clinical outcome of the phage therapy. This study also showed that phage-anti-phage synergism had a significant impact on the clinical outcome of the patient and had a little impact on those who showed a weak immune response to phage treatment [117]. The theoretical model proposed by Leung and Weitz has shown the synergistic evidence of coexisting phage and immune response in eliminating the infections [118]. The available data on phage therapy indicates that the phages are highly safe and efficient to treat bacterial infections. But with the on-going research on immunological aspects and other immune response after phage administration in the immunocompetent individual will open the hidden concepts behind phage therapy. In future, these research data will bring evidences for the efficacy and safety of phage therapy in various individuals.

**Pharmacodynamic and Pharmacokinetic Aspect of Phage Therapy**

When considering phage therapy, one must consider the treatment choices such as route of administration, possible side effects, and standard pharmacological aspects. Before any drug is administered in humans, the pharmacodynamic (PD) and pharmacokinetic (PK) aspects of the molecule have to be assessed. An imbalanced effect of either PK or PD might result in an inefficient treatment outcome [119]. Pharmacology of phage therapy involves the specificity of the phages against a target pathogen, efficiency and efficacy of phage therapy, route of administration and distribution of phages to the other organs of the body, emergence of bacterial resistant mutants, rate of adsorption, and multiplicity of infection. All these therapeutic outcomes should be considered before a phage is prescribed for human use [120, 121].

## Phage Pharmacodynamics

Pharmacodynamic deals with the effect and the mechanism of the drug inside the living system. Phage infection is initiated by the random kinetic of the phage that recognizes the bacterial receptors [122]. Several points have to be taken into consideration such as the dosage (limited by the size of the phage) and route of administration, *etc.* Phage tends to be more of an easier translocating type than antibiotics. Many studies have shown that irrespective of the route of administration of the phage, the presence of high titer of phage were noted in multiple organs in distant location [123]. Phage dosing may differ between the patients based on the site of infection and the condition of the patient [124]. As phages are self-replicating most of the clinicians don't consider them, but maintaining the killing titre is important to bring out effective therapy. Based on the dosage and formulations, pharmacodynamic might hold either a negative or a positive impact on the body [125]. Phage preparations should be ensured for purity as they can induce immune responses. This can be avoided by the removal of endotoxin, selection of virulent phage, and checking for the presence of virulent or toxin genes in the phage genome.

The host range determines the functionality of the phage in bringing up the bactericidal effect on the various clones of the bacteria. The ability of the phage to kill the bacteria can be divided into two types: 1. Transductive host range, in which bacteria can take up the phage DNA, but doesn't merely cause lysis of the bacteria. 2. Bactericidal host range, in which bacteria is killed upon the phage multiplication cycle [126]. The phage density obtained during the treatment is very crucial to bring out the effective treatment strategy and the titer of phage to be given during the treatment [127]. The bacterial physiological activity plays a major role in determining the effect of phage burst size. A study conducted by Ramesh *et al.* 2019 has shown that phage plaque morphology changes or differs in different bacteriological media, which is due to the different composition of the media, which directly affect the bacterial physiological activity there by altering the phage multiplication and burst size [128]. The bacteria that are having less physiological activity tend to produce smaller phage burst size when compared to the others. In such cases, the physician will recommend an additional dosage to boost up the therapy irrespective of the initial dose [129]. These effects can be overcome by defining the phage activity before taking them for the therapy. But most of the laboratory output of the phage might not match the *in-situ* performance, which can be due to the different body environment and chemical makeup of the system. During those situations, phage formulation plays a commending role. The use of phage cocktails and the use of phage encapsulation for prolonged therapy has become a choice of treatment [113]. The phage cocktail enables the use of phages against multiple infections and applying them in extended geographical locations. These phages are transported either in a dry form or in an encapsulated form as a bead (hydrogel or alginate) [130]. These methods of transportation increase the shelf-life of the phages without any loss in the titer. Phage encapsulation helps in delayed and slow release of phages that improves the phage availability at the infection site for a prolonged period. This also gives stability to the acidic condition of stomach acids and thermal stability. Abdelsattar *et al.*, 2019 showed that phage encapsulated in alginate bead remained viable for 8 weeks at 4°C without any change in the titer. They also reported the stability of the phages at low pH that helped in sustaining the phages over a longer duration, which shows that encapsulation has an enhanced and significant pharmacodynamic effect [131].

**Phage Pharmacokinetics**

Phage pharmacokinetics deals with the movement of phages (drug) within the body. Phage has a different mechanism of kinetics when compared to antibiotics. Phages are made of proteins and found to be much larger in size than the antibiotics or chemicals. Phages have numerous advantages in the distribution and circulation within the human body. Phage pharmacokinetics is divided into four major types as absorption, distribution, excretion, and metabolism (Fig. 7) [132].

**Adsorption**

Adsorption of the phage is determined by the kinetics of bacteria and phage in the circulation. The random collision of phage and bacteria brings about the phage to get adsorbed onto the bacterial receptors [133]. The smaller phages (only tailed phages are chosen for therapy) are said to have a higher dynamic than the larger phages, thus small phages are the primary choice of phage therapy. The smaller sized phage tends to show increased burst size and shorter latency period.

**Distribution**

The route of phage administration influences the distribution of phages. The different route includes topical, oral, intraperitoneal, intramuscular, and subcutaneous. The route of administration is determined by the site of infection.

Intravenous delivery of phages is found to be more efficient method of phage dispersal [134]. The oral route is a complicated choice for phage delivery as they have to travel through acidic conditions. But experimentally, those phages that can survive acidic conditions are chosen for therapy. Adsorption of phages to the circulatory system was found to be very less when phages are given orally but this is an effective method for gastrointestinal infections [120]. The effect of phage translocation and induction of anti-phage has been observed to be high when administered orally. Tropical delivery is another method of phage application, a preferred method for the skin and other localized wound infections. The inhalant formulated for lung infections is as equally effective as the topical application [135]. The bacterial biofilm at the implant site is a very tedious infection to treat. The movement and distribution of phages within biofilm matrices is considered to be an obstacle for the biofilm treatment. Recent studies have shown that the phages have adapted the ability to overcome this effect by producing depolymerase that degrades the biofilm, thereby, increasing their chances of invading the bacteria. The blood-brain barrier is often a site of challenge for the drug distribution. It was though that the phage being larger than a chemical molecule can be hard to pass the blood-brain barrier but studies have shown that phages can cross the blood-brain barrier within 1 hr of their administration [85].

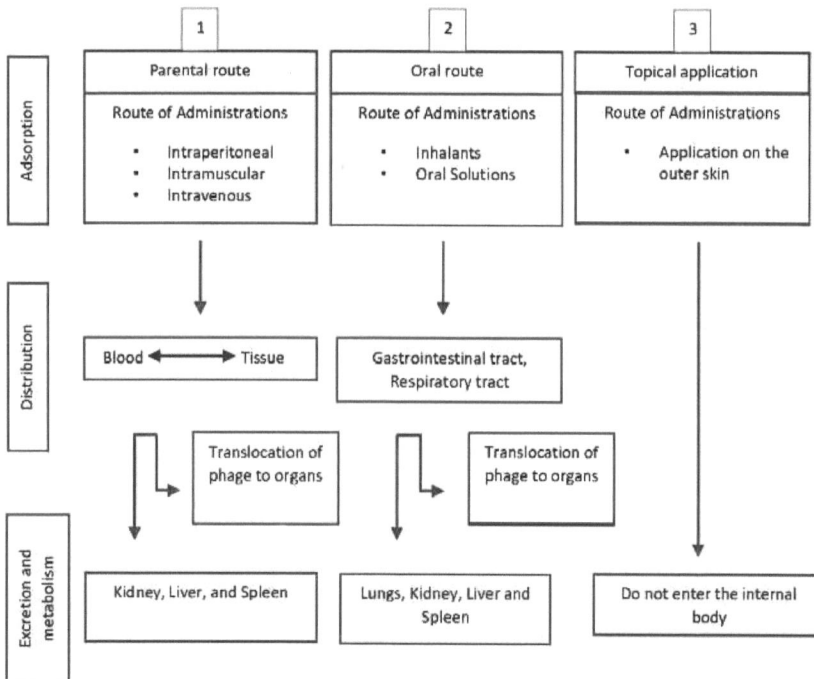

**Fig. (7).** Pharmacokinetics of phages administered through different routes (route of administration).

## Excretion and Metabolism

Phages that enter the body undergo multiplication and replicate to produce progeny phage particles, and the cycle continues until the host bacterium exhausted. These therapeutic phages are eliminated from our body through various mechanisms mostly accompanied by the kidneys [125]. A study by Tiwari *et al.*, showed that a median half-life of phage was 4.5 hours after the administration [136]. The half-life or the inactivation of phages can be improved by encapsulating the phages such as in hydrogels. This method also had improved phage protection against acidic environment with slow and prolonged dispersion within the body [137]. Renal clearance results in the secretion of drugs or any molecules by flushing them in the urine. Numerous bacteria are found to be present in the urine culture [138]. Phages were also detected in the urine of humans. Most of the research outcome found that phage clearance by the renal system showed a variation among the individuals based on the age and other external factors. The urine titre of the phages was found to be less than the blood. Apart from the kidneys, liver and spleen are also found to filter out the circulating phages. A study by Inchley *et al.*, 1969 showed that phage accumulated more in the liver than any other organ [139].

## APPLICATION OF PHAGE THERAPY AGAINST BACTERIAL INFECTIONS

### Phage Therapy for Wound Infections

Wound infections are often prone to bacterial infections due to its exposure to opportunistic pathogens, including multidrug-resistant (MDR) bacteria. Unlike gut which holds the vast majority of microorganisms ($\sim 10^4$), the skin acts as a physical barrier, resisting microorganisms and potential toxins while retaining moisture and nutrients inside the body [140, 141] (Grice & Segre, 2011; Hooper, 2001). Clinically wounds occurs due to external damage to intact skin caused by surgery, burns, chemicals or wounds due to chronic diabetic ulcers. Proper wound care is needed for an infection-free closure before the exposed subcutaneous provides a favourable substrate for the bacteria to take over. Typically, endogenous Gram-positive bacteria initially colonize the wound site but later replaced by antibiotic-susceptible Gram-negative bacteria. The use of broad-spectrum antibiotics to treat these infections tends to favour exogenous nosocomial pathogens, which are generally antibiotic-resistant bacteria such as methicillin-resistant *S. aureus* (MRSA), vancomycin-resistant enterococci and extended-spectrum β-lactamase (ESBL)-producing Gram-negative bacteria which are difficult to treat [142, 143]. Phage therapy against wound (burn) infections started way back in 1970 when Shera applied phage lysate impregnated gauze against *S. aureus* at the wound site of a young man and successfully healed the burn wounds [144]. In recent years, phage formulations and delivery methods for applications of phages for the treatment of acute and chronic wound infections were developed.

McVay *et al.*, 2007 reported a single dose of a cocktail consisting of three different *P. aeruginosa* phages could significantly reduce the mortality of thermally injured *P. aeruginosa*-infected mice. The intraperitoneal administration of the phage cocktail could increase the survival of burn wound *P. aeruginosa* infected mice [145].

Merabishvili *et al.*, 2009 used a phage cocktail that consisted of two *Pseudomonas* phages (14/1 and PNM) and one *Staphylococcus* phage (ISP) for the treatment of *P. aeruginosa* and *S. aureus* infections in burn wound patients. The cocktail showed large host range specifically against burn-wound bacterial isolates and were successful in the treatment of eight patients suffering from infected burn wounds without any adverse effects [146].

Malik and Chhibber, 2009 proved that bacteriophage KO1 isolated from the environment could be protective against *K. pneumoniae* induced mouse model of burn wound infection. The phage treatment substantially decreased the bacterial load of blood, peritoneal lavage, and lung tissue [147].

Seema *et al.*, 2009 evaluated the therapeutic potential of five *Klebsiella* phages (Kpn5, Kpn12, Kpn13, Kpn17, and Kpn22) administered intraperitoneally as individual phages or in cocktail against *K. pneumoniae* B5055 infected mice model of burn wounds. The phages were able to rescue the burned and infected mice with a single dose at 24h post-infection with a percentage survival ranging from 80-97%. The phage Kpn5 was effective and showed highest percentage survival (97.22%) comparable with the mice treated with a cocktail. The phages also reduced the bacterial load in blood, peritoneal fluid, lungs, and skin significantly [148]. In another study, they applied the phage Kpn5 topically at the wound site after establishment of infection. The phage loaded in 3% hydrogel provided a high level of protection (63% survival) at day 7 when compared with antimicrobial agents such as silver nitrate (5%) or gentamicin (1000 mg l$^{-1}$) for the same burn wound model. Silver nitrate and gentamycin treated mice found to have survival rates of 57 and 53%, respectively [149].

Meurice *et al.*, 2012 claimed hydroxyapatite (HA) and β-tricalcium phosphate (β-TCP) ceramics loaded with phages could be used as a prophylactic agent during bone surgery to prevent bacterial infection. HA and β-TCP were commonly used as bone substitutes in orthopaedic and dental surgery and encounters bacterial infection in the surgical wound. The λ phage-loaded β-TCP and HA were able to release the phages for at least 6 days and exhibit antibacterial activity against *E. coli* similar to that of antibiotics proving phages could replace antibiotics in prophylactic treatments [150].

Diabetic foot infections caused by MRSA are often linked with an increased risk of amputations. MRSA accounts for 43% of diabetic foot infections and the colonized wounds show delayed healing. Antibiotics such as tigecycline, vancomycin and linezolid were commonly used for treating diabetic foot infections; however, strains resistant to these antibiotics have already emerged in hospital and community settings. Chibber *et al.*, 2013 demonstrated that combination therapy using bacteriophage MR-10 and linezolid was effective in eliminating MRSA from diabetic foot infections. MRSA induced acute hindpaw infection in alloxan induced diabetic BALB/c mice was completely resolved by the combination therapy 7 days post-infection and the bacterial load was negligible at the site of infection. The phage-antibiotic combination has the advantage to check the development of linezolid-resistant mutants, therefore, presents a new alternative treatment option for MRSA infections in diabetic patients [151].

*Acinetobacter baumannii* is another opportunistic pathogen emerged as an important infective agent among the foot ulcers in diabetic individuals. The emergence of pan-drug resistant strains demands the need for the control of *Acinetobacter* infections. A study carried out by Mendes *et al.*, 2013 indicated that bacteriophage cocktail (*S. aureus* phages F44/10 and F125/10, *P. aeruginosa* phages F770/05 and F510/08, and *A. baumannii* phage F1245/05) when applied topically improved the healing potential in debrided-infected wounds of diabetic Wistar rats which were infected with *S. aureus, P. aeruginosa*, and *A. baumannii*. A round wound was inflicted in the interscapular region of the rats and were infected with *S. aureus, P. aeruginosa*, or *A. baumannii* and phage cocktail was administered post 4, 5 and 8 days of wounding and debridement. Swabs were collected from the wound site to assess bacterial counts in the region and the phage cocktail treatment significantly reduced the bacterial load and accelerated the wound closure in the foot ulcers [152].

In another study, Shivaswamy *et al.*, 2015 studied the therapeutic potential of bacteriophages that were specific against MDR *A. baumannii* and used to treat wound infection in diabetic rats. Similar to previous study, the wounds were debrided before the application of the bacteriophages at the wound site. Phages significantly reduced the duration of epithelialization and increased the percentage of wound contraction in the excision wound model in rats indicating phage prophylaxis against experimental MDR *A. baumannii* infections in rats [153].

Basu *et al.*, 2015 described the efficacy of bacteriophages in clearing MDR *P. aeruginosa* biofilms generated on sterile catheter sections in a mouse wound model. Biofilm-laden catheter sections were implanted in subcutaneous pockets at the back of albino mice and phage cocktail (10 µL of $10^7$ phage forming units/mL) were injected at the subcutaneous pocket for 10 days. The results showed that in the phage treated mice, the bacterial load decreased significantly compared to the control groups, and a significant rise in the phage counts also were observed, indicating the ability of the phages to destroy the MDR *P. aeruginosa* biofilm created in the wound [154].

Regeimbal *et al.*, 2016 employed a five-member phage cocktail against *A. baumannii* in a mouse full-thickness dorsal infected wound model. The cocktail lowers the bacterial population in the wound, prevents the spread of infection and necrosis to the surrounding tissues, and decreases infection-associated morbidity in mice. One of the phages in the cocktail was isolated using *A. baumannii* AB5075 as a host from environmental samples and designated as AB-Army1. AB-Army1 infection leads to loss-of-capsule phenotype in *A. baumannii* AB5075 strain and it is designated as AB5075P. The AB5075P strain was used to isolate the other phages AB-Navy1, AB-Navy2, AB-Navy3 and AB-Navy4 of the cocktail. Interestingly, the cocktail works in a co-operative manner where upon AB-Army1 infection the strain becomes sensitive to other phages results in effective killing. This study is an example of design and execution of intelligent phage cocktails to control emergent strains during the treatment [62].

Chadha *et al.*, 2017 compared the therapeutic efficacy of free phage cocktail and liposome entrapped phage cocktail in solving the course of burn wound infection in mice. Liposomes improved the bioavailability of the entrapped phages and released the phages at steady rate and regular intervals, thus maintaining high phage titer for a longer duration. Hence, animals treated with liposome entrapped phage cocktail (LCP) showed significant reduction in bacterial counts in much shorter period as compared to free phage cocktail in the study [66]. Similarly liposome entrapped phages improved wound healing of *S. aureus*-induced excision wound infection in diabetic mice in another study from the same lab [155].

*E. coli*, another most common colonizer and prolific biofilm-forming bacteria which is difficult to control and eliminate from infected wounds. Study by Oliveira *et al.*, 2018 demonstrated the synergistic action of chestnut honey and *E. coli* and *P. aeruginosa* phages vB_EcoS_CEB_EC3a and vB_PaeP_PAO1-D, respectively, against *E. coli* biofilms in an *ex vivo* (porcine skin) wound model. Mono- or dual-species biofilms of *E. coli* and *P. aeruginosa* formed on porcine skins were targeted using chestnut honey and the phage combination resulted in bacterial elimination. The antibacterial efficacy of the combination may be due to honey's ability to damage the bacterial cell membrane and penetrating the biofilm matrix, thereby, promoting and enhancing the subsequent phage infections [156].

Non-healing wounds are a great challenge to surgeons as they may occasionally result in amputation of the affected part. A chronic wound usually results due to the infection by antibiotic-resistant bacteria and subsequent biofilm formation. Gupta *et al.*, 2019 studied a total of 20 patients with chronic non-healing wound infections. They were either not responding to conventional local debridement or antibiotic therapy. A customized bacteriophage cocktail was selected and topically applied over the wounds resulted in significant improvement in wound healing, and no signs of infection clinically and microbiologically after 3 to 5 doses of topical phage applications [157].

Nanofibers loaded with the bacteriophage were tested as wound dressings for their antibacterial activity and enhanced wound healing. Sarhan and Azzazy (2017) loaded honey, polyvinyl alcohol, chitosan (HPCS) nano-fibrous mats with bacteriophages to show the wound-healing ability in a mice wound model. Among the nanofibers developed in the study, the HPCS-bacteriophage nanofibers showed broad-spectrum antibacterial activity, enhanced biocompatibility, wound closure rate and accelerated the wound healing [158].

Kaur *et al.*, 2019 established a novel wound dressing model consisting of Polyvinyl Alcohol (PVA) – Sodium Alginate (SA) hybrid hydrogel membrane for topical delivery of bacteriophages. The PVA-SA blend has combined advantages of high hydrophilicity, biocompatibility, membrane- forming ability, biodegradability, protein adsorption ability and non-toxic. The PVA-SA hydrogel was poured onto sterile cotton gauze and bacteriophages were loaded onto the surface of the membrane. The phage loaded PVA-SA membrane adhering to burn wound in mice was found to be most effective in preventing bacterial infection as well as enhancing the healing of infected wound tissue [159].

Recently, Kifelew *et al.*, 2020 studied the efficacy of phage cocktail AB-SA01 in diabetic mouse wound infections caused by multidrug-resistant *S. aureus*. The cocktail consists of three *S. aureus* phages (J-Sa36, Sa83, and Sa87) which has undergone two phase I clinical trials, in treatment of multidrug-resistant (MDR) *S. aureus* infections. Topical application of phage cocktail AB-SA01 leads to complete wound healing, evident by the decrease in wound size during and after the course of treatment [160].

## Phage Therapy for Cystic Fibrosis

Cystic fibrosis (CF) is a lethal genetic disease that is characterized by the obstruction of the respiratory airways resulting in chronic infection leading to progressive deterioration of lung function. *S. aureus* plays an important role in causing infections in infants, whereas, *Pseudomonas* sp. contributes to infection in adults. Typically, patients with CF survive with antibiotics for an extended period of time; however, the emergence of MDR bacterial strains leads to increased mortality. Classically, oral cephalosporins, ampicillin, and combination of trimethoprim/sulfamethoxazole were prescribed for mild infections and for severe cases ticarcillin, carbenicillin, the ureidopenicillins, and the aminoglycosides are prescribed [161]. *P. aeruginosa* is the most common pathogen responsible for hospital-acquired bacterial pneumonia as well as ventilator-associated pneumonia. But next to *S. aureus*, *Pseudomonas* is also the causative agent of CF in patients [162, 163]. *P. aeruginosa* colonizes in the lung sites in CF and typically produces biofilm which make them insensitive to antibiotics. Lytic bacteriophages could be the answer to treat these antibiotic resistant bacteria because the depolymerase enzymes produced by lytic bacteriophages has the ability to degrade the biofilms and lyse the *P. aeruginosa* at the site of infection [164].

Debarbieux *et al.*, 2008 isolated the bacteriophage PAK-P1 using the bioluminescent *P. aeruginosa* PAK strain which was obtained from French cystic fibrosis strain collection centre, Grenoble, France. Bioluminescent *P. aeruginosa* strain was used to infect mice to record a real-time view of the lung infection, thus the spatial and temporal development of infections was monitored. Bacteriophages when applied intranasally, able to reduce the bacterial load in the phage-treated mice compared to the non-phage treated mice. The bacteriophage also prevented the development of infection when treated empirically at the site of infection [165].

Morello *et al.*, 2011 demonstrated bacteriophage therapy on *P. aeruginosa* CF strains in mouse lung infection model. The PAK-P3 bacteriophage was able to establish a moderate infection in *P. aeruginosa* CHA strain, MDR mucoid strain isolated from a CF patient of Grenoble hospital, France. Two doses of P3-CHA bacteriophage administered intranasally to mice infected with CHA strain showed improved survival as compared with phage untreated group [166].

*Burkholderia cenocepacia* is another opportunistic and life-threatening pathogen for CF patients. The infection can lead to acute pulmonary diseases and sepsis ("cepacia syndrome") or chronic infection characterized by an accelerated decline in lung function in patients. Seed and Dennis, 2009 validated that the phage therapy increases the survival of *Galleria mellonella* larvae infected with *B.*

*cenocepacia* strains K56-2 and C6433 that had spread epidemically among patients with CF. Phage KS4-M rescued *B. cenocepacia*-infected *G. mellonella* larvae from death when the larvae received a single injection of phage immediately after the infection. Similar results were obtained with three more phages KS12, KS14, and DC1 [167].

Carmody *et al.*, 2010 showed the efficacy of phage therapy using mice model with *B. cenocepacia* pulmonary infection. Phage BcepIL02 was administered either by intranasal inhalation or intraperitoneal injection in mice at a multiplicity of infection of 100 and bacterial densities in lungs were determined after 48 h. Intraperitoneal injection of phage BcepIL02 resulted in a significant reduction in lung bacterial density post-administration [168].

Alemayehu *et al.*, 2012 evaluated the efficacy of two bacteriophages φNH-4 (myovirus) and φMR299-2 (podovirus) isolated from a local wastewater treatment plant to kill the *P. aeruginosa* in the murine lung or biofilm on a pulmonary cell line. They examined the ability of φNH-4 and φMR299-2 phages to clear 24 h-old biofilms of *P. aeruginosa* CF isolates NH57388A or MR299 on cystic fibrosis bronchial epithelial, CFBE41o- cells. The phage titres increased almost 2 log units during the 24 h period, confirming the significant phage replication occurred at the biofilm site and staining proved the considerable destruction to the biofilm structure. They also examined the ability of phages to kill *Pseudomonas in situ* in the lungs of infected 8-week-old female BALB/c mice. Phage treatment prevented the growth and reduced the bacterial load to a non-detectable levels during the 6 h treatment in (mice) lungs [169].

Lynch *et al.*, 2013 identified three putative intact prophages in the CF clinical isolate *B. cenocepacia* H111 genome. One of the prophages, φH111-1 showed extremely broad host-range and is predicted to use lipopolysaccharide (LPS) as a receptor. φH111-1 was tested against 13 strains of *B. cenocepacia* acquired from the University of Alberta Hospital Cystic Fibrosis Clinic, Canada [170].

Kamal and Dennis, 2015 observed phage-antibiotic synergy (PAS) when phages KS12 and KS14 were tested for PAS with ampicillin, ceftazidime, ciprofloxacin, kanamycin, levofloxacin, meropenem, minocycline, piperacillin, and tetracycline against *B. cenocepacia* strains C6433 and K56-2 cells. The phages showed an increase in plaque size in the presence of different concentrations of antibiotics indicating that the antibiotics stimulate lytic phage activity. *G. mellonella* larvae was infected with *B. cenocepacia* and treated with a combination of phage and antibiotics, meropenem and minocycline. The larvae were rescued with a sharp decrease in the mortality from 80% to 22% when treated with meropenem alone or 67% when treated with phage KS12 alone at 48 h post-infection. Similarly, the larval mortality decreased from 76% to 31% when phage KS12 plus minocycline were treated together [77].

Sahota *et al.*, 2015 examined the efficacy of bacteriophages against Liverpool Epidemic Strain (LES), the most common cystic fibrosis-related *P. aeruginosa* clone in the UK. All the 84 phenotypically variable isolates of the LES were tested for susceptibility against two phages, PELP20 and PELI40, and the phages killed 98% of the tested strains [171].

Olszak *et al.*, 2015 isolated bacteriophages from a natural wastewater treatment plant (irrigated fields) located in Wroclaw, Poland, against CF *P. aeruginosa* strains isolated from patients. A total of 123 *P. aeruginosa* isolates were used to test the phage lytic potency including 121 clinical CF isolates from the collection of the Prague CF Centre. Two phages PA5oct and KT28 from the collection exhibited high antibacterial potency, with 55% and 68% of the isolates tested respectively [172].

Pabary *et al.*, 2015 tested *P. aeruginosa* PAO1 and other strains that were isolated from the sputa of adult in-patients with CF at the Royal Brompton Hospital, London against three novel bacteriophage cocktails; cocktail 1 (*P. aeruginosa* 24, *P. aeruginosa* 25, and *P. aeruginosa* 7), cocktail 2 (*P. aeruginosa* 39, *P. aeruginosa* 67, *P. aeruginosa* 77, and *P. aeruginosa* 119) and cocktail 3 (*P. aeruginosa* 3, *P. aeruginosa* 6, *P. aeruginosa* 10, *P. aeruginosa* 32, and *P. aeruginosa* 37). When tested against the clinical isolates, phage cocktail 1 was active against the 5 clinical isolates, while the cocktails 2 and 3 infected only 3 out of the 5 tested isolates/strains. Adult BALB/c mice were anesthetized by isoflurane inhalation and were infected with PAO1 and clinical isolates by intranasal sniffing for phage treatment. Phage cocktails (20 µl) were administered intranasally 24 h post-infection, or 48 h pre-infection and bronchoalveolar lavage fluid (BALF) were assessed at various times for infective burden and inflammation. No bacteria were cultured from BAL fluid from any phage-treated mice indicating the clearance of bacteria in the mice lungs. The prophylactic administration of bacteriophages 48 h prior to bacterial infection resulted in undetected levels of bacteria in the BAL fluid at 24 h post-infection [173].

Waters *et al.*, 2017 used a natural respiratory inhalation route of infection and showed that phage therapy is an effective treatment against chronic *P. aeruginosa* lung infections. *P. aeruginosa* LESB65 isolated from patients with CF were infected intranasally that readily establishes chronic infection in the murine lung. Phage was administered both at 24 or 36 h post-infection and in both the cases; complete clearance of *P. aeruginosa* from the lungs was achieved. They further extended the treatment gap and administered phage post 6 days after infection and found phage therapy was again highly effective against the established 6-day lung infection with significant clearance of bacteria from the lungs of 70% mice tested.

This is the first study reporting the efficacy of phage therapy up to 7 days post-infection in a mice model [174].

Shiley *et al.*, 2017 employed a human lung *in vitro* model using A549 cell line to study the efficacy of bacteriophages PEV2 and DMS3. The A549 cells were infected with *P. aeruginosa* PAO1 cells before addition of PEV2 and DMS3 phages. The phage DMS3 was extremely effective at protecting the A549 cells from *P. aeruginosa*, whereas, phage PEV2 was less effective [175].

Forti *et al.*, 2018 demonstrated that a 6 phage cocktail composed of four novel phages (PYO2, DEV, E215 and E217) with the phages (PAK_P1 and PAK_P4) was able to lyse *P. aeruginosa* strains collected from Italian cystic fibrosis (CF) patients. The phage cocktail had a distinct host range, with no individual phage being able to lyse all strains but lysed 30 out of 40 Italian cystic fibrosis (CF) strains *in vitro*. The phage cocktail cleared the biofilm formed on glass slides and cured *P. aeruginosa* acute respiratory infection in a mouse model by reducing the respiratory bacterial burden at 48 h and achieving a 100% survival rate [68].

Lin *et al.*, 2018 investigated synergistic effect of phage PEV20 with 1/4 MIC of five different antibiotics, ciprofloxacin, amikacin, aztreonam, colistin and tobramycin against *P. aeruginosa* strains FADD1-PA001 and JIP865 isolated from the sputum samples of CF patients. Ciprofloxacin-phage PEV20 exhibited synergy to eliminate the *Pseudomonas* infection [176].

*Achromobacter xylosoxidans*, recognized as an emerging nosocomial pathogen that is capable of colonizing and causing infections in CF patients. *Achromobacter* colonization among CF patients may be acquired either from the environment or *via* cross-contamination and horizontal transmission between patients. Hoyle *et al.*, 2018 described the case of cystic fibrosis complicated with a chronic MDR *A. xylosoxidans* lung infection treated with phage cocktail at the Eliava phage therapy centre, Tbilisi, Georgia. The phage cocktail was administered both *via* inhalation using a compression nebulizer (once daily) and orally (twice daily), for 20 days. The patients subjective conditions significantly improved, cough reduced and lung function improved to 80% after phage treatment [177].

Cafora *et al.*, 2019 applied phage therapy for the treatment of *P. aeruginosa* PAO1 infections in a CF zebrafish model. PAO1 infection was performed in zebrafish embryos at 48 h post-infection and injected the phage cocktail in the yolk sac of PAO1-infected embryos. They observed that lethality of PAO1 infection reduced from 70% to 42 % and to 38 % in early to late injections. Further studies on the effects of combining phages and antibiotics (100 µg/ml ciprofloxacin and phage cocktail) in embryos reduced the lethality of infection. This study showed that zebra fish model could be adapted in future to test CF treatment [178].

Law *et al.*, 2019 described the use of phage therapy in a 26-year-old CF patient awaiting lung transplantation. Use of intravenous phages along with systemic antibiotics for 100 days resulted in no recurrence of pseudomonal pneumonia and CF exacerbation. The patient underwent successful bilateral lung transplantation nine months post-therapy [179].

Gainey *et al.*, 2020 presented a clinical case of a 10-year-old female CF patient, infected with a Pan-drug resistant *Achromobacter* sp. A patient was given a phage-antibiotic combination to restore baseline pulmonary function. By combining the phage, Ax2CJ45Φ2, with cefiderocol and meropenem/ vaborbactam, *Achromobacter* sp. was eliminated from the site of infection which was confirmed using the collected sputum samples after eight weeks and 16 weeks post-treatment [180].

Non-tuberculosis mycobacteria (NTM), *Mycobacterium abscessus* have recently been emerged as important pathogen among CF patients. Dedrick *et al.*, 2019 reported a successful case study of 15-year-old cystic fibrosis patient with a disseminated *M. abscessus* infection which was treated with three-phage cocktail following bilateral lung transplantation. The patient was chronically infected with *P. aeruginosa* and *M. abscessus* subspecies *massiliense* and had been on anti-NTM treatment for 8 years. She was treated with a phage cocktail of three mycobacteriophages Muddy, BPs33ΔHTH-HRM10 and recombinant ZoeJc, intravenously every 12 h for at least 32 weeks. The phage treatment was well tolerated throughout without significant side effects and over the next six months the patient improved clinically with gradual healing of surgical wound and skin lesions, improved lung function, liver function and gaining weight. This was the first therapeutic use of phages for human mycobacterial infection [15].

**Phage Therapy for Urinary Tract Infections**

Urinary tract infections (UTIs) are considered as one of the common bacterial diseases in adults [181, 182]. UTIs affect women of all ages more often than men and >50% of women experience UTIs at least once in their life time. Treatment for UTIs usually involve antibiotics and currently, trimethoprim, sulfamethoxazole, cotrinoxazole, ciprofloxacin, ampicillin, second or third generation cephalosporins, carbapenems and nitrofurantoin were the most recommended and frequently prescribed antibiotics. The widespread and uncontrolled use of antibiotics resulted in the increasing antibiotic resistance and emergence of multi-drug resistant (MDR) and extensively drug-resistant (XDR) uropathogens [183, 184]. Various uropathogens were linked with UTIs including *E. coli* (~85%), *Proteus mirabilis, K. pneumoniae, Staphylococcus saphrophyticus, S. aureus,* group B *Streptococcus, Enterobacter* and *Enterococcus* sp., and *Candida* sp. Uropathogenic *E. coli* strains (UPECs) are the most dominant etiologic agent constituting 80–90% of bacteria that cause urinary infections during pregnancy [182, 185]. Increasing resistance and biofilm-formation makes the uropathogens almost untreatable using the antibiotics, therefore, alternative approaches for the prevention and treatment of UTIs is required. Phage therapy has a potential to eliminate uropathogens within the urinary tract. Lytic bacteriophages, genetically modified or engineered phages, phage-derived enzymes, phage-antibiotic combination makes the innovative and promising therapeutic options [183, 186].

Nishikawa *et al.*, 2008 examined the possibility of phage therapy for UTIs caused by the UPEC strains. An uropathogenic *E. coli* strain ECU5 was injected transurethrally into the mouse bladder to establish *E. coli*-caused UTI model in mice. Two phages, T4 and KEP10 were studied for its antibacterial activity. Administration of these phages into the peritoneal cavity decreased the mortality of mice inoculated transurethrally with a UPEC strain [187].

Sillankorva *et al.*, 2010 investigated the use of lytic bacteriophages against *E. coli* adhered to urothelium. *E. coli* was adhered to epithelial cell line from human bladder (TCC-SUP) for 2 h to form urothelium in this study. The T1-like bacteriophage caused nearly a 45% reduction of the bacterial population after 2 h of treatment to the adhered cells indicating a viable alternative to antibiotics in controlling urothelium-adhered bacteria [188].

*Cronobacter* sp. is a rare but dangerous opportunistic pathogen among UTI pathogens. Tóthová *et al.*, 2011 showed the efficiency of *Cronobacter*-specific phages on renal colonization in a UTI mice model. Urinary tract infection was induced by transurethral application of *Cronobacter turicensis* strain in mice and *Cronobacter*-specific phages were administered intraperitoneally. The phages reduced the number of *Cronobacter* colonies in the kidney by 70% indicating its effect in the prevention of ascending renal infection in murine UTI model [189].

Chibeu *et al.*, 2012 demonstrated the ability of bacteriophages to degrade UPEC biofilms. They studied 253 UTI *E. coli* isolates for their ability to form biofilm and found only 42 produced biofilms in microtiter plate. The lytic activity of three phages, ACG-C91, ACG-C40 and ACG-M12, were tested against the biofilm forming *E. coli* UTI isolates which showed 80.5% of the isolates were infected by at least one phage [190].

*Proteus mirabilis*, a hospital acquired opportunistic pathogen which forms dense crystalline biofilms on catheter surfaces in long-term catheterized patients often leading to serious clinical complications. Nzakizwanayo *et al.*, 2016 evaluated the potential of phage therapy to control *P. mirabilis* infection and prevent catheter blockage, using three phage (ΦRS1-PmA, ΦRS1-PmB, and ΦRS3-PmA) cocktail. A single dose of the phage cocktail extended the time taken for catheters to block, significantly and completely prevented the catheter blockage [191].

Melo *et al.*, 2016 developed a phage cocktail to control *P. mirabilis* catheter-associated UTIs. Two novel virulent phages, vB_PmiP_5460 (podovirus) and vB_PmiM_5461 (myovirus) were isolated and tested for its ability to infect *Proteus* strains. Their spectrum of activity against a collection of *Proteus* sp. was 16/26 and 26/26, respectively. Foley catheters either phage cocktail coated or non-coated were used to mimic the renal urinary catheters to study the effect of phages on a continuous biofilm model. Phage-coating led to the reduction in the biofilm population leading to significant reductions at 96 h and 168 h, representing the tendency of the phage cocktail to reduce *P. mirabilis* biofilms [192].

Leitner *et al.*, 2017 designed a randomized, placebo-controlled, double-blind clinical trial to assess the efficacy and safety of intravesical bacteriophage treatment for UTIs in patients undergoing transurethral resection of the prostate. Commercially available Pyo bacteriophage was used in this study. Patients planned for transurethral resection of the prostate are screened for UTIs and only patients with Pyo bacteriophage sensitive bacterial infection was included in the study. The patients received 20 ml of phages at 12 h interval (twice a day) for 7 days through suprapubic catheter and asked to retain the phage for 30-60 min in the bladder. No evidence of bacteria after 7 days post-phage treatment showed successful phage application [193].

Yazdi *et al.*, 2018 applied a combination of a lytic bacteriophage, vB_PmiS-TH and ampicillin to demonstrate the lytic activity of the phage-antibiotic combination against *P. mirabilis* planktonic cells and biofilms. Phage vB_PmiS-TH along with sub-MIC of ampicillin (8 μg/mL) had a synergetic effect on planktonic *P. mirabilis* reflected by the decrease in bacterial load and also had a great potential in the prevention of biofilm formation. The phage at an MOI of 100 along with the antibiotic (246 μg/mL) removed 93% of the biofilm cells after 24 h [194].

Gu *et al.*, 2019 isolated novel bacteriophage, vB_EcoP-EG1 from local waste water which showed lytic activity against planktonic and biofilm forming UPECs.

The phage appeared to be relatively specific and infected 10 out of 21 clinical multi-drug resistant UPEC strains. The phage also affected biofilm formation of *E. coli* MG1655 and clinical strain 390G7 when tested in microtiter wells [195].

Moradpour *et al.*, 2020 determined the synergistic effect of a naturally isolated phage and ampicillin against *E. coli* O157. The phage, gT0E.co-MGY2 added to the microbial lawn of bacteria in modified antibiotic disk diffusion test, the bacteria altered its phenotype from resistant to sensitive and significantly enhanced the synergistic effect of ampicillin in liquid culture [196].

Grygorcewicz *et al.*, 2020 assessed the effects of phage cocktail and antibiotic combination against *A. baumannii* in a human urine model. *A. baumannii* AB20 was MDR causing UTIs and is a strong biofilm producer. A phage cocktail containing five phages namely, Aba-1, Aba-2, Aba-3, Aba-4, and Aba-6, isolated from different environmental samples collected in the West Pomeranian Region, Poland. The growth medium was replaced with human filtered urine to establish a human urine model and the bacteria were able to produce biofilm in the urine. The phage cocktail was used in combination with antibiotics, ciprofloxacin, trimethoprim/ sulfamethoxazole, gentamicin, tobramycin, imipenem and meropenem, resulted in a significant reduction of biofilm biomass [197].

Rostkowska *et al.*, 2020 presented a case study of a 60-year-old patient who experienced several episodes of UTI due to multi-drug resistant ESBL-producing *K. pneumoniae* after kidney transplantation. Phage therapy was applied on the experimental basis for 29 days which controlled the *K. pneumoniae* infection eventually leading to full recovery [198].

## Phage Therapy for Respiratory Infections

Antibiotic resistance has also become a major problem in the treatment of infections of the respiratory system. In recent years, substantial efforts have been made towards therapeutic application of bacteriophages as an alternative over conventional antibiotics for respiratory infections [199]. Inhalation of high concentration of bacteriophages was considered as the successful route of administration of phages and often considered advantageous because the treatment of bacterial lung infections with conventional antibiotic therapy may not get access to the heavy bacterial load in deeper lung, whereas bacteriophages which has the ability to replicate at the site of infection can access and eliminate the bacteria [135, 200]. *P. aeruginosa, S. aureus, K. pneumoniae, A. baumannii, B. cepacia complex (BCC), and M. tuberculosis* are the most common bacterial species often associated with lung infections. Inhaled phages were reported in the 1960s when Delacoste successfully treated refractory cough using phage cocktail administered through a nebulizer. Hoeflmayr also reported the successful use of nebulized phage cocktail in treating patients with chronic bronchitis [135, 199, 200].

Chhibber *et al.*, 2008 employed a mouse model of *K. pneumoniae*-associated lobar pneumonia and studied the efficacy of phage SS. Mice were challenged with *K. pneumoniae* intranasally, whereas, the phage was administered intraperitoneally. The study demonstrated the timing of starting the phage therapy after initiation of infection significantly contributes towards the success of the treatment. Immediate administration of phages after bacterial challenge rescued 100% mice while prophylactic treatment (3 h prior to intranasal bacterial challenge) provided significant protection of infected mice. Phage administration after 6 h post-bacterial challenge rendered the phage treatment failure [201].

Shen *et al.*, 2012 isolated eight phages from hospital sewage and prepared a phage cocktail (φkm18p, φTZ1 and φ314) that could lyse 15 clinical isolates with phage φkm18p being the most effective. They also evaluated the therapeutic potential of phage φkm18p using human lung epithelial cells A549 as an experiment model. Human lung epithelial cells inoculated with *A. baumannii* KM18 strain were completely killed while phage φkm18p increased the survival rate after 24 h of incubation [202].

Drilling *et al.*, 2014 demonstrated that phages has the potential to treat *S. aureus* infection and biofilm-formation in chronic rhinosinusitis patients. A phage cocktail, CT-SA was found active against 62 of 66 (94%) clinical isolates tested and significantly reduced the biofilm mass produced by the clinical isolates [203]. Similarly, the cocktail demonstrated anti-biofilm activity against *P. aeruginosa* isolates in chronic rhinosinusitis patients. Fong *et al.*, 2017 studied phage cocktail, CT-SA against *P. aeruginosa* isolates from chronic rhinosinusitis patients (CRS) patients with and without CF. CT-PA treatment significantly reduced biofilm *in vitro* at 24 and 48 h post-treatment by a median of 76% at 48 h.

Takemura-Uchiyama *et al.*, 2014 described phage therapy against *S. aureus* induced lethal lung-derived septicemia in mice. The phage S13 used in this study can efficiently lyse hospital-acquired MRSA strains *in vitro*. An intraperitoneal administration of phage S13 at 6 h post-infection significantly reduced the severity of infection and recovered 70% of mice from mortality [204].

Semler *et al.*, 2015 showed aerosol phage therapy has better efficacy than phage treatment by intraperitoneal injections. In this study, *B. cenocepacia* infections in mice were established by a jet nebulizer attached to a nose-only inhalation device (NOID). Following infection, phage KS12 was delivered simultaneously through NOID and intraperitoneal injection. Significant decrease in the bacterial load was observed in mice lungs of NOID-delivered KS12 as compared to intraperitoneal administration of phages after 2 days of infection. The reason might be, intranasally delivered phages localized to the alveolar macrophages, whereas i.p.-delivered phages localized to the perivascular areas and the alveolar septa in mice [204].

Singla *et al.*, 2015 packaged phage KPO1K2 within liposomes for intraperitoneal administration in a mouse model of *K. pneumonia*-associated lobar pneumonia. The liposome-entrapped phages (LEP) were able to survive for long duration in the circulation in comparison with free phages, when administered intraperitoneally. Free phages were able to prevent the bacterial infection when administered 3 h or 6 h prior to bacterial challenge, but failed to prevent the infection at 24 h prior treatment. LEP provided complete protection given 6 h, 24 h, or 48 h prior to bacterial challenge. LEP administration after 6 h, 24 h, 48 h, and 72 h of infection resulted in significant reductions in bacterial load in mice lungs indicating the extended effect of entrapped phages [205].

Wang *et al.*, 2016 evaluated the therapeutic efficacy of intranasal treatment of phages in *A. baumannii*-induced pneumonia in mice model. Mice administered with *A. baumannii* by intranasal treatment were allowed to establish pneumonia and the phage vB_AbaM-IME-AB2 isolated from the hospital sewage was introduced intranasally 1 h post-infection. Treatment with the lytic bacteriophage significantly reduced the bacterial load in mouse lung and *A. baumannii* was eradicated after 144 h post-treatment [206].

Chang *et al.*, 2017 produced highly stable spray dried phage formulations for treatment of *P. aeruginosa* lung infection containing trehalose or lactose and leucine as excipients. Seven phages were tested for bactericidal activity against 90 *P. aeruginosa* strains for the assessment of host-range and three phages, namely PEV1, PEV20 and PEV61 showed high killing efficiency over 70% of *P. aeruginosa* clinical and MDR strains tested [207].

Chang *et al.*, 2018 assessed the bactericidal activities of phage dry-powder formulations against MDR *P. aeruginosa* in a mouse lung infection model. An inhalable dry-powder phage formulation was produced by spray drying highly purified phage PEV20 with lactose and leucine. The lung infection in mice was established by intratracheal administration of *P. aeruginosa* FADDI-PA001 strain. The infected mice were treated with 2 mg of the phage powder using a dry-powder insufflator 2 h post-bacterial challenge. At 24 h post-phage treatment, the bacterial load in the lungs were decreased significantly indicating the possibility of pulmonary delivery of phage PEV20 dry-powder formulation for the treatment of lung infection [208].

Jeon *et al.*, 2019 studied the efficacy of bacteriophage treatment against carbapenem-resistant *A. baumannii* in a mouse model of acute pneumonia. The *A. baumannii* phage Bϕ-R2096 isolated from sewage water at the University Hospital in South Korea was used in this study. The phage Bϕ-R2096 increased the survival rates of mice for 12 days post-infection with bacterial clearance in the lungs observed on day 3 post-infection suggesting phage Bϕ-R2096 as an alternative agent to control *A. baumannii* infections in acute pneumonia [209].

In another study, Jeon and Yong (2019) evaluated the efficacy of two bacteriophages in mouse acute pneumonia model infected with extensively drug-resistant *P. aeruginosa*. Bϕ-R656 and Bϕ-R1836 exhibited broad host-range lysing 18 and 14 out of 28 XDR *P. aeruginosa* strains. Treatment with Bϕ-R656 and Bϕ-R1836 enhanced the survival of mice with pneumonia after 12 days of infection and significantly decreased the bacterial load in the lungs [210].

Prazak *et al.*, 2019 tested the efficacy of cocktail of four phages namely 2003, 2002, 3A, and K, for the treatment of ventilator-associated pneumonia due to MRSA in rats. Treatment with phages increased the survival of the animal from 0% to 58% with reduced bacterial burdens in the lungs [211]. All the clinical cases are tabulated, (Table **3**).

**Table 3. Summary of the pre-clinical and clinical studies performed to evaluate the efficacy of phage therapy against bacterial infections.**

| Phage(s) | Target(s) | Model | Treatment for | Delivery | References |
|---|---|---|---|---|---|
| Pa1, Pa2 and Pa11 | *P. aeruginosa* | Mouse | Burn wounds | Intraperitoneal | [145] |
| 14/1 and PNM, ISP | *P. aeruginosa, S. aureus* | Human | Burn wounds | Topical | [146] |
| KO1 | *K. pneumoniae* | Mouse | Burn wounds | Subcutaneous/ Intraperitoneal | [147] |
| Kpn5, Kpn12, Kpn13, Kpn17, and Kpn22 | *K. pneumoniae* | Mouse | Burn wounds | Intraperitoneal | [148] |
| Kpn5 loaded in 3% hydrogel | *K. pneumoniae* | Mouse | Burn wounds | Topical | [149] |
| λ phage-loaded β-TCP and HA | *E. coli* | Bone repair | Burn wounds | Suspension | [150] |
| MR-10 | MRSA | Mouse | Diabetic foot infections | Subcutaneous | [151] |
| F44/10 and F125/10 F770/05 and F510/08 F1245/05 | *S. aureus, P. aeruginosa, A. baumannii* | Rat | Diabetic wounds | Topical | [152] |
| *Acinetobacter* phage | MDR *A. baumannii* | Rat | Diabetic wounds | Topical | [153] |

*(Table 3) cont.....*

| Phage(s) | Target(s) | Model | Treatment for | Delivery | References |
|---|---|---|---|---|---|
| Phage cocktail | MDR P. aeruginosa | Mouse | Surgical Wound | Subcutaneous | [154] |
| AB-Army1, AB-Navy1, AB-Navy2, AB-Navy3 and AB-Navy4 | A. baumannii | Galleria mellonella, Mouse | Surgical wounds | Intraperitoneal | [62] |
| Liposome entrapped phage cocktail (LCP) | S. aureus | Mouse | Burn wounds | Intraperitoneal | [66, 155] |
| vB_EcoS_CEB_EC3a, vB_PaeP_PAO1-D | E. coli, P. aeruginosa | Ex Vivo (porcine skin) | Wounds | Topical | [156] |
| Phage cocktail | E. coli, S. aureus, P. aeruginosa. | Human | Non-healing wounds | Topical | [157] |
| Phage PS1 loaded HPCS-BV nanofibers | MDR P. aeruginosa | Mouse | Wounds | Topical | [158] |
| Phage MR10 loaded in PVA-SA hydrogel | MRSA | Mouse | Wounds | Topical | [159] |
| J- Sa36, Sa83, and Sa87 (phage cocktail AB-SA01) | MDR S. aureus | Mouse | Wounds | Topical | [160] |
| PAK-P1 | P. aeruginosa | Mouse | Cystic Fibrosis | Intranasal | [165] |
| PAK-P3 | P. aeruginosa | Mouse | Cystic Fibrosis | Intranasal | [166] |
| KS4-M, KS12, KS14, and DC1 | B. cenocepacia | Galleria mellonella | Cystic Fibrosis | Intraperitoneal | [167] |
| BcepIL02 | B. cenocepacia | Mouse | Cystic Fibrosis | Intranasal/ Intraperitoneal | [168] |
| φNH-4 and φMR299-2 | P. aeruginosa | Ex Vivo (CFBE41o-cells) Mouse | Cystic Fibrosis | Intranasal | [169] |
| φH111-1 | B. cenocepacia | 13 Clinical isolates | Cystic Fibrosis | Suspension | [170] |
| KS12 and KS14 | B. cenocepacia | Galleria mellonella | Cystic Fibrosis | Intraperitoneal | [77] |
| PELP20, PELI40 | P. aeruginosa Liverpool Epidemic Strain (LES) | 84 Clinical isolates | Cystic Fibrosis | Suspension | [171] |

*(Table 3) cont.....*

| Phage(s) | Target(s) | Model | Treatment for | Delivery | References |
|---|---|---|---|---|---|
| PA5oct, KT28 | *P. aeruginosa* | 121 Clinical isolates | Cystic Fibrosis | Suspension | [172] |
| Cocktail 1 (*P. aeruginosa* 24, 25, and 7), Cocktail 2 (*P. aeruginosa* 39, 67, 77, and 119), Cocktail 3 (*P. aeruginosa* 3, 6, 10, 32, and 37) | *P. aeruginosa* | Mouse | Cystic Fibrosis | Intranasal | [173] |
| PELP20 | *P. aeruginosa* | Mouse | Cystic Fibrosis | Intranasal | [174] |
| PEV2 and DMS3 | *P. aeruginosa* | *Ex Vivo* (A549 cells) | Cystic Fibrosis | Suspension | [175] |
| PYO2, DEV, E215, E217, PAK_P1 and PAK_P4 | *P. aeruginosa* | Mouse | Cystic Fibrosis | Intranasal | [68] |
| PEV20 | *P. aeruginosa* | Clinical isolates | Cystic Fibrosis | Suspension | [176] |
| Two *Achromobacter* phages | MDR *A. xylosoxidans* | Human | Cystic Fibrosis | Intranasal/ Oral | [177] |
| vB_PaeP_PYO2, vB_PaeP_DEV, vB_PaeM_E215, vB_PaeM_E217 | *P. aeruginosa* | Zebra fish | Cystic Fibrosis | Injected in the yolk sac | [178] |
| AB-PA01 | *P. aeruginosa* | Human | Pneumonia and Cystic Fibrosis | Intravenous | [179] |
| Ax2CJ45Φ2 | PDR *Achromobacter* sp. | Human | Cystic fibrosis | Intravenous | [180] |
| Mycobacteriophage Muddy, BPs33ΔHTH-HRM10 and recombineered ZoeJc | *M. abscessus* | Human | Cystic fibrosis | Intravenous | [15] |
| T4, KEP10 | Uropathogenic *E. coli* (UPECs) | Mouse | Urinary Tract Infections | Intraperitoneal | [187] |

*(Table 3) cont.....*

| Phage(s) | Target(s) | Model | Treatment for | Delivery | References |
|---|---|---|---|---|---|
| T1- like bacteriophage | *E. coli* | *Ex Vivo* (TCC-SUP) | Urinary Tract Infections | Suspension | [188] |
| *Cronobacter*-specific phages | *Cronobacter turicensis* | Mouse | Urinary Tract Infections | Intraperitoneal | [189] |
| ACG-C91, ACG-C40, ACG-M12 | *E. coli* | 253 Clinical isolates | Urinary Tract Infections | Suspension | [190] |
| ΦRS1-PmA, ΦRS1-PmB, ΦRS3-PmA | *P. mirabilis* | Foley catheters | Urinary Tract Infections | Suspension | [191] |
| vB_PmiP_5460, vB_PmiM_5461 | *P. mirabilis* | Foley catheters | Urinary Tract Infections | Foley catheters coated phages | [192] |
| Pyo bacteriophage | Pyo bacteriophage sensitive bacteria | Human | Urinary Tract Infections | Intravesical | [193] |
| vB_PmiS-TH | *P. mirabilis* | Clinical isolates | Urinary Tract Infections | Suspension | [194] |
| vB_EcoP-EG1 | Uropathogenic *E. coli* (UPECs) | 21 Clinical isolates | Urinary Tract Infections | Suspension | [55] |
| gT0E.co-MGY2 | *E. coli* | Clinical isolate | Urinary Tract Infections | Suspension | [196] |
| Aba-1, Aba-2, Aba-3, Aba-4, and Aba-6 | *A. baumannii* | Human urine model | Urinary Tract Infections | Suspension | [197] |
| Custom phages | ESBL-producing *K. pneumoniae* | Human | Urinary Tract Infections | Intrarectal | [198] |
| SS | *K. pneumoniae* | Mouse | Pneumonia | Intranasal | [201] |
| φkm18p, φTZ1 and φ314 | *A. baumannii* | *Ex Vivo* (A549 cells) | Respiratory tract infections | Suspension | [202] |
| CT-SA | *S. aureus* | 66 Clinical isolates | Chronic rhinosinusitis | Suspension | [203] |
| CT-PA | *P. aeruginosa* | 47 Clinical isolates | Chronic rhinosinusitis | Suspension | [212] |

*(Table 3) cont.....*

| Phage(s) | Target(s) | Model | Treatment for | Delivery | References |
|---|---|---|---|---|---|
| S13 | MRSA | Mouse | Lung Septicemia | Intraperitoneal | [204] |
| KS12 | *B. cenocepacia* | Mouse | Respiratory tract infections | Intraperitoneal/Intranasal | [213] |
| Liposome-entrapped KPO1K2 | *K. pneumoniae* | Mouse | Pneumonia | Intraperitoneal | [205] |
| vB_AbaM-IME-AB2 | *A. baumannii* | Mouse | Pneumonia | Intranasal | [206] |
| PEV1, PEV20 and PEV61 | *P. aeruginosa* | 90 Clinical isolates | Lung infections | Suspension | [207] |
| PEV20 | *P. aeruginosa* | Mouse | Lung infections | Intranasal | [208] |
| Bϕ-R2096 | *A. baumannii* | Mouse | Pneumonia | Intranasal | [209] |
| Bϕ-R656 and Bϕ-R1836 | *P. aeruginosa* | Mouse | Pneumonia | Intranasal | [210] |
| 2003, 2002, 3A, and K | *S. aureus* | Rat | Pneumonia | Intravenous | [211] |

## CHALLENGES AND THE FUTURE OF PHAGE THERAPY

Phage therapy was renewed in late 1990s to tackle the problem of antibiotic resistance and some important developments and discoveries were made thereafter (Fig. **1**). But there are major therapeutic hurdles that need to be addressed before phage therapy is applied at large scale for human use. A) Lack of proper regulatory guidelines: both government and private firms are not ready to invest in phage therapy research (& development) because of the uncertainty in the use of phage therapy, which is directly linked to companies' profit. There are concerns over the existing 'regulatory pathways' and 'intellectual property (IP) protection' [214]. Though the application of phage-based products is approved for food protection, there are no proper guidelines for human applications [215]. For phages to be used as a therapeutic tool to treat human infections, drug regulatory agencies require researchers to demonstrate the safety and efficacy of phage therapy. Another concern is over the collection and the distribution of phages at the time of treatment and the concept of creating phage libraries or phage banks has to be considered [216]. In order to use the proper and certified phage stocks in therapy, governments can setup phage laboratories that will certify the phage stocks after careful examination. Only certified phage stocks can be used for treatment [217]. B) Selection of obligate lytic phages for treatment: Phages are available in natural environments but selecting appropriate 'obligate' lytic phages for therapy is necessary for treatment success. Appropriate administration of phages to the patients (based on the nature of infection) is another critical procedure during treatment [31]. There is no standard administration procedure for phage therapy and phages are known to have narrow-spectrum activity (antibiotics are broad-spectrum) that might hinder the therapeutic outcome. C) Public awareness: From the patients point-of-view 'phages are viruses' therefore getting patient consent will be challenging. Mainly because of the lack of enough clinical trials and uncertainty about the risks associated with phage treatment.

Phages can be used in 'One-Health approach' which recognizes the health of humans, animals and our environment as one or interlinked. Phages are used to control or kill the bacteria, therefore, under One Health approach phages can be used to treat human diseases [14], animal infections [218], to preserve food products [219] and in the environment for wastewater treatment [220, 221]. Thus, bacteriophages can be used in different settings to control the bacterial growth that eventually reduces the overuse of antibiotics and eliminates the dissemination of antibiotic-resistant bacteria.

Synthetic phages are produced by cell-free systems that enable the on-site production of phages for therapeutic purpose [222]. There are considerable advantages in using synthetic phages that includes, a) there is no need to maintain phage banks and exchange of bacterial or phage isolates can be avoided, b) on-site production of phages during major bacterial outbreaks, c) phages can be easily produced against complicated bacteria or bacteria that are causing lethal diseases using phage genomic sequences or metagenomic data [223, 224], and d) phage preparations will be free of endotoxins. Another approach is the use of endolysins as antibacterial agents. Endolysins are phage-derived enzymes that can hydrolyse bacterial outer membranes and are part of the phage life cycle where the new progeny phages are released by degrading the bacterial outer membranes (lysis from inside). Though the use of endolysins is largely studied against Gram-positive bacteria, more studies are needed to prove their efficacy against Gram-negative bacteria [225]. Endolysins are proteins that can readily combine with other antibacterials (antibiotics) to fight against (pathogenic) bacteria and found to have multiple applications in various sectors. Studies on endolysins and their application are growing at a faster rate and detailed reports can be found elsewhere [226, 227]. Recently, efforts have been made to study the efficacy of encapsulated bacteriophages for phage therapy [113]. Encapsulated phage preparations were found to have very good efficacy to cure bacterial infections in the studied animal models [70, 155]. In future, genetically engineered phage techniques are also emerging to advance and broaden the phage therapy applications [228]. Lots of efforts have been made by the researchers to improve the phage preparations for therapy (toxin-free) and standard techniques should be formulated to ease the difficulty in preparing phages for therapeutic applications

[229]. The future of phage therapy looks promising and clinical trials are necessary to prove their efficacy. Despite phages are considered as one of the alternatives to antibiotics (MDR infections), it is not appropriate to say that 'phages will replace antibiotics' as a whole.

## CONCLUSION

Comparing to the pre-antibiotic era (in the 1920s), the post-antibiotic era (after 2000) has brought substantial improvement in the knowledge and understanding about the bacteriophages and their therapeutic applications. Still, enormous efforts are needed from the government and funding agencies to support phage therapy research and to setup global phage banks and implement personalised phage therapy. Clinical trials including challenge studies should be undertaken with government support so that untreatable (antibiotics) bacterial infections can be treated using phage cocktails. More accurate information is required to prove the safety and efficacy of phage therapy, and also to understand the risks and benefits that are associated with phage therapy.

## CONSENT FOR PUBLICATION

Not applicable.

## CONFLICT OF INTEREST

The author declares no conflict of interest, financial or otherwise.

## ACKNOWLEDGEMENTS

Declared none.

## REFERENCES

[1]    Gordillo Altamirano FL, Barr JJ. Phage therapy in the postantibiotic era. Clin Microbiol Rev 2019; 32(2): e00066-18.
[http://dx.doi.org/10.1128/CMR.00066-18] [PMID: 30651225]

[2]    Podolsky SH. The evolving response to antibiotic resistance (1945–2018). Palgrave Commun 2018; 4: 124.
[http://dx.doi.org/10.1057/s41599-018-0181-x]

[3]    Manohar P, Shanthini T, Ayyanar R, *et al.* The distribution of carbapenem- and colistin-resistance in Gram-negative bacteria from the Tamil Nadu region in India. J Med Microbiol 2017; 66(7): 874-83.
[http://dx.doi.org/10.1099/jmm.0.000508] [PMID: 28671537]

[4]    Manohar P, Loh B, Leptihn S. Will the overuse of antibiotics during the coronavirus pandemic accelerate antimicrobial resistance of bacteria? 2020.
[http://dx.doi.org/10.1097/IM9.0000000000000034]

[5]    Hankin ME. The bactericidal action of the waters of the Jamuna and Ganges rivers on Cholera microbes. Ann. Inst. Pasteur 10:511–523 (1896). Bacteriophage 2011; 1: 117-26.

[http://dx.doi.org/10.4161/bact.1.3.16736]

[6]     Emmerich R, Löw O. Die künstliche Darstellung der immunisirenden Substanzen (Nucleasen-Immunproteïdine) und ihre Verwendung zur Therapie der Infectionskrankheiten und zur Schutzimpfung an Stelle des Heilserums. Zeitschrift Für Hyg Und Infekt 1901; 36: 9-28.
[http://dx.doi.org/10.1007/BF02141216]

[7]     Summers WC. History of phage research and phage therapy. Phages 2014; pp. 1-17.

[8]     d'Herelle FS. ur un microbe invisible antagoniste des bacilles dysentériques. C R Acad Sci Paris. 1917;165:173–5. Ann Pasteur Institute 1896; III: 300.

[9]     Bruynoghe RAMJ. Essais de thérapeutique au moyen du bacteriophage. CR Soc Biol 1921; 85: 1120-1.

[10]    F D. Essai de traîtement de la peste bubonique par le bactériophage. Press Med 1925; 33

[11]    d'Herelle F, Malone RH LM. Studies on Asiatic cholera. Studies on Asiatic Cholera. Mem No 14 1930

[12]    Wright A, Hawkins CH, Anggård EE, Harper DR. A controlled clinical trial of a therapeutic bacteriophage preparation in chronic otitis due to antibiotic-resistant Pseudomonas aeruginosa; a preliminary report of efficacy. Clin Otolaryngol 2009; 34(4): 349-57.
[http://dx.doi.org/10.1111/j.1749-4486.2009.01973.x] [PMID: 19673983]

[13]    Jault P, Leclerc T, Jennes S, et al. Efficacy and tolerability of a cocktail of bacteriophages to treat burn wounds infected by Pseudomonas aeruginosa (PhagoBurn): a randomised, controlled, double-blind phase 1/2 trial. Lancet Infect Dis 2019; 19(1): 35-45.
[http://dx.doi.org/10.1016/S1473-3099(18)30482-1] [PMID: 30292481]

[14]    Schooley RT, Biswas B, Gill JJ, et al. Development and use of personalized bacteriophage-based therapeutic cocktails to treat a patient with a disseminated resistant acinetobacter baumannii infection. Antimicrob Agents Chemother 2017; 61(10): e00954-17.
[http://dx.doi.org/10.1128/AAC.00954-17] [PMID: 28807909]

[15]    Dedrick RM, Guerrero-Bustamante CA, Garlena RA, et al. Engineered bacteriophages for treatment of a patient with a disseminated drug-resistant Mycobacterium abscessus. Nat Med 2019; 25(5): 730-3.
[http://dx.doi.org/10.1038/s41591-019-0437-z] [PMID: 31068712]

[16]    Manohar P, Loh B, Athira S, et al. Secondary bacterial infections during pulmonary viral disease: phage therapeutics as alternatives to antibiotics? Front Microbiol 2020; 11: 1434.
[http://dx.doi.org/10.3389/fmicb.2020.01434] [PMID: 32733404]

[17]    Lin DM, Koskella B, Lin HC. Phage therapy: An alternative to antibiotics in the age of multi-drug resistance. World J Gastrointest Pharmacol Ther 2017; 8(3): 162-73.
[http://dx.doi.org/10.4292/wjgpt.v8.i3.162] [PMID: 28828194]

[18]    Koskella B, Meaden S. Understanding bacteriophage specificity in natural microbial communities. Viruses 2013; 5(3): 806-23.
[http://dx.doi.org/10.3390/v5030806] [PMID: 23478639]

[19]    Labrie SJ, Samson JE, Moineau S. Bacteriophage resistance mechanisms. Nat Rev Microbiol 2010; 8(5): 317-27.
[http://dx.doi.org/10.1038/nrmicro2315] [PMID: 20348932]

[20]    Koskella B, Brockhurst MA. Bacteria-phage coevolution as a driver of ecological and evolutionary processes in microbial communities. FEMS Microbiol Rev 2014; 38(5): 916-31.
[http://dx.doi.org/10.1111/1574-6976.12072] [PMID: 24617569]

[21]    Pawluk A, Davidson AR, Maxwell KL. Anti-CRISPR: discovery, mechanism and function. Nat Rev Microbiol 2018; 16(1): 12-7.
[http://dx.doi.org/10.1038/nrmicro.2017.120] [PMID: 29062071]

[22]    The Bacteriophages. NY, USA: Oxford Univ Press New York 2006; p. 746.

[23]     Simmonds P, Adams MJ, Benkő M, *et al.* Consensus statement: Virus taxonomy in the age of metagenomics. Nat Rev Microbiol 2017; 15(3): 161-8.
[http://dx.doi.org/10.1038/nrmicro.2016.177] [PMID: 28134265]

[24]     Adriaenssens E, Brister JR. How to name and classify your phage: An informal guide. Viruses 2017; 9(4): 70.
[http://dx.doi.org/10.3390/v9040070] [PMID: 28368359]

[25]     Dion MB, Oechslin F, Moineau S. Phage diversity, genomics and phylogeny. Nat Rev Microbiol 2020; 18(3): 125-38.
[http://dx.doi.org/10.1038/s41579-019-0311-5] [PMID: 32015529]

[26]     Lavigne R, Seto D, Mahadevan P, Ackermann H-W, Kropinski AM. Unifying classical and molecular taxonomic classification: analysis of the Podoviridae using BLASTP-based tools. Res Microbiol 2008; 159(5): 406-14.
[http://dx.doi.org/10.1016/j.resmic.2008.03.005] [PMID: 18555669]

[27]     Jamalludeen N, Johnson RP, Friendship R, Kropinski AM, Lingohr EJ, Gyles CL. Isolation and characterization of nine bacteriophages that lyse O149 enterotoxigenic *Escherichia coli.* Vet Microbiol 2007; 124(1-2): 47-57.
[http://dx.doi.org/10.1016/j.vetmic.2007.03.028] [PMID: 17560053]

[28]     Demerec M, Fano U. U F. Bacteriophage-resistant mutants in *Escherichia coli.* Genetics 1945; 30(2): 119-36.
[PMID: 17247150]

[29]     Adriaenssens EM, Sullivan MB, Knezevic P, *et al.* Taxonomy of prokaryotic viruses: 2018-2019 update from the ICTV Bacterial and Archaeal Viruses Subcommittee. Arch Virol 2020; 165(5): 1253-60.
[http://dx.doi.org/10.1007/s00705-020-04577-8] [PMID: 32162068]

[30]     Adriaenssens EM, Wittmann J, Kuhn JH, *et al.* Taxonomy of prokaryotic viruses: 2017 update from the ICTV Bacterial and Archaeal Viruses Subcommittee. Arch Virol 2018; 163(4): 1125-9.
[http://dx.doi.org/10.1007/s00705-018-3723-z] [PMID: 29356990]

[31]     Loc-Carrillo C, Abedon ST. Pros and cons of phage therapy. Bacteriophage 2011; 1(2): 111-4.
[http://dx.doi.org/10.4161/bact.1.2.14590] [PMID: 22334867]

[32]     Wienhold S-M, Lienau J, Witzenrath M. Towards inhaled phage therapy in western europe. Viruses 2019; 11(3): 295.
[http://dx.doi.org/10.3390/v11030295] [PMID: 30909579]

[33]     Nordström K, Forsgren A. Effect of protein A on adsorption of bacteriophages to Staphylococcus aureus. J Virol 1974; 14(2): 198-202.
[http://dx.doi.org/10.1128/JVI.14.2.198-202.1974] [PMID: 4277011]

[34]     Stummeyer K, Schwarzer D, Claus H, Vogel U, Gerardy-Schahn R, Mühlenhoff M. Evolution of bacteriophages infecting encapsulated bacteria: lessons from *Escherichia coli* K1-specific phages. Mol Microbiol 2006; 60(5): 1123-35.
[http://dx.doi.org/10.1111/j.1365-2958.2006.05173.x] [PMID: 16689790]

[35]     Destoumieux-Garzón D, Duquesne S, Peduzzi J, *et al.* The iron-siderophore transporter FhuA is the receptor for the antimicrobial peptide microcin J25: role of the microcin Val11-Pro16 β-hairpin region in the recognition mechanism. Biochem J 2005; 389(Pt 3): 869-76.
[http://dx.doi.org/10.1042/BJ20042107] [PMID: 15862112]

[36]     Lu M-J, Henning U. Superinfection exclusion by T-even-type coliphages. Trends Microbiol 1994; 2(4): 137-9.
[http://dx.doi.org/10.1016/0966-842X(94)90601-7] [PMID: 8012757]

[37]     Kliem M, Dreiseikelmann B. The superimmunity gene sim of bacteriophage P1 causes superinfection exclusion. Virology 1989; 171(2): 350-5.

[http://dx.doi.org/10.1016/0042-6822(89)90602-8] [PMID: 2763457]

[38]   Garvey P, Hill C, Fitzgerald GF. The lactococcal plasmid pnp40 encodes a third bacteriophage resistance mechanism, one which affects phage dna penetration. Appl Environ Microbiol 1996; 62(2): 676-9.
[http://dx.doi.org/10.1128/AEM.62.2.676-679.1996] [PMID: 16535245]

[39]   Pingoud A, Fuxreiter M, Pingoud V, Wende W. Type II restriction endonucleases: structure and mechanism. Cell Mol Life Sci 2005; 62(6): 685-707.
[http://dx.doi.org/10.1007/s00018-004-4513-1] [PMID: 15770420]

[40]   Bujnicki JM. Molecular phylogenetics of restriction endonucleases. Restrict Endonucleases 2004; pp. 63-93.
[http://dx.doi.org/10.1007/978-3-642-18851-0_3]

[41]   Bair CL, Rifat D, Black LW. Exclusion of glucosyl-hydroxymethylcytosine DNA containing bacteriophages is overcome by the injected protein inhibitor IPI*. J Mol Biol 2007; 366(3): 779-89.
[http://dx.doi.org/10.1016/j.jmb.2006.11.049] [PMID: 17188711]

[42]   Atanasiu C, Su TJ, Sturrock SS, Dryden DT. Interaction of the ocr gene 0.3 protein of bacteriophage T7 with EcoKI restriction/modification enzyme. Nucleic Acids Res 2002; 30(18): 3936-44.
[http://dx.doi.org/10.1093/nar/gkf518] [PMID: 12235377]

[43]   Barrangou R, Fremaux C, Deveau H, *et al.* CRISPR provides acquired resistance against viruses in prokaryotes 2007.
[http://dx.doi.org/10.1126/science.1138140]

[44]   Horvath P, Barrangou R. CRISPR/Cas, the immune system of bacteria and archaea. Science 2010; 327: 167-70.

[45]   Azam AH, Tanji Y. Bacteriophage-host arm race: an update on the mechanism of phage resistance in bacteria and revenge of the phage with the perspective for phage therapy. Appl Microbiol Biotechnol 2019; 103(5): 2121-31.
[http://dx.doi.org/10.1007/s00253-019-09629-x] [PMID: 30680434]

[46]   Ofir G, Melamed S, Sberro H, *et al.* DISARM is a widespread bacterial defence system with broad anti-phage activities. Nat Microbiol 2018; 3(1): 90-8.
[http://dx.doi.org/10.1038/s41564-017-0051-0] [PMID: 29085076]

[47]   IJ M. Host-parasite interactions: recent developments in the genetics of abortive phage infections. New Biol 1: 230-6. n.d.

[48]   Doron S, Melamed S, Ofir G, *et al.* Systematic discovery of antiphage defense systems in the microbial pangenome. Science 2018; 359(6379): eaar4120.
[http://dx.doi.org/10.1126/science.aar4120]

[49]   Smith HW, Huggins MB. Successful treatment of experimental *Escherichia coli* infections in mice using phage: its general superiority over antibiotics. J Gen Microbiol 1982; 128(2): 307-18.
[http://dx.doi.org/10.1099/00221287-128-2-307] [PMID: 7042903]

[50]   Smith HW, Huggins MB, Shaw KM. The control of experimental *Escherichia coli* diarrhoea in calves by means of bacteriophages. J Gen Microbiol 1987; 133(5): 1111-26.
[http://dx.doi.org/10.1099/00221287-133-5-1111] [PMID: 3309177]

[51]   Zhvania P, Hoyle NS, Nadareishvili L, Nizharadze D, Kutateladze M. Phage therapy in a 16-year-old boy with netherton syndrome. Front Med (Lausanne) 2017; 4: 94.
[http://dx.doi.org/10.3389/fmed.2017.00094] [PMID: 28717637]

[52]   Oechslin F. Resistance development to bacteriophages occurring during bacteriophage therapy. Viruses 2018; 10(7): 351.
[http://dx.doi.org/10.3390/v10070351] [PMID: 29966329]

[53]   Wright RCT, Friman V-P, Smith MCM, Brockhurst MA. Resistance evolution against phage

combinations depends on the timing and order of exposure. MBio 2019; 10(5): e01652-19. [http://dx.doi.org/10.1128/mBio.01652-19] [PMID: 31551330]

[54]	Chan BK, Abedon ST, Loc-Carrillo C. Phage cocktails and the future of phage therapy. Future Microbiol 2013; 8(6): 769-83. [http://dx.doi.org/10.2217/fmb.13.47] [PMID: 23701332]

[55]	Gu J, Liu X, Li Y, *et al.* A method for generation phage cocktail with great therapeutic potential. PLoS One 2012; 7(3): e31698. [http://dx.doi.org/10.1371/journal.pone.0031698] [PMID: 22396736]

[56]	O'Flynn G, Ross RP, Fitzgerald GF, Coffey A. Evaluation of a cocktail of three bacteriophages for biocontrol of *Escherichia coli* O157:H7. Appl Environ Microbiol 2004; 70(6): 3417-24. [http://dx.doi.org/10.1128/AEM.70.6.3417-3424.2004] [PMID: 15184139]

[57]	Tanji Y, Shimada T, Yoichi M, Miyanaga K, Hori K, Unno H. Toward rational control of *Escherichia coli* O157:H7 by a phage cocktail. Appl Microbiol Biotechnol 2004; 64(2): 270-4. [http://dx.doi.org/10.1007/s00253-003-1438-9] [PMID: 13680205]

[58]	Abedon ST, Kuhl SJ, Blasdel BG, Kutter EM. Phage treatment of human infections. Bacteriophage 2011; 1(2): 66-85. [http://dx.doi.org/10.4161/bact.1.2.15845] [PMID: 22334863]

[59]	Pirnay J-P, De Vos D, Verbeken G, *et al.* The phage therapy paradigm: prêt-à-porter or sur-mesure? Pharm Res 2011; 28(4): 934-7. [http://dx.doi.org/10.1007/s11095-010-0313-5] [PMID: 21063753]

[60]	Międzybrodzki R, Borysowski J, Weber-Dąbrowska B, *et al.* Clinical aspects of phage therapy. Adv Virus Res 2012; 83: 73-121. [http://dx.doi.org/10.1016/B978-0-12-394438-2.00003-7] [PMID: 22748809]

[61]	Górski A, Międzybrodzki R, Weber-Dąbrowska B, *et al.* Phage therapy: combating infections with potential for evolving from merely a treatment for complications to targeting diseases. Front Microbiol 2016; 7: 1515. [http://dx.doi.org/10.3389/fmicb.2016.01515] [PMID: 27725811]

[62]	Regeimbal JM, Jacobs AC, Corey BW, *et al.* Personalized therapeutic cocktail of wild environmental phages rescues mice from acinetobacter baumannii wound infections. Antimicrob Agents Chemother 2016; 60(10): 5806-16. [http://dx.doi.org/10.1128/AAC.02877-15] [PMID: 27431214]

[63]	Aslam S, Yung G, Dan J, Reed S, LeFebvre M, Logan C, *et al.* Bacteriophage treatment in a lung transplant recipient. J Heart Lung Transplant 2018; 37: S155-6. [http://dx.doi.org/10.1016/j.healun.2018.01.376]

[64]	Khawaldeh A, Morales S, Dillon B, *et al.* Bacteriophage therapy for refractory Pseudomonas aeruginosa urinary tract infection. J Med Microbiol 2011; 60(Pt 11): 1697-700. [http://dx.doi.org/10.1099/jmm.0.029744-0] [PMID: 21737541]

[65]	Yu L, Wang S, Guo Z, *et al.* A guard-killer phage cocktail effectively lyses the host and inhibits the development of phage-resistant strains of *Escherichia coli.* Appl Microbiol Biotechnol 2018; 102(2): 971-83. [http://dx.doi.org/10.1007/s00253-017-8591-z] [PMID: 29150707]

[66]	Chadha P, Katare OP, Chhibber S. Liposome loaded phage cocktail: Enhanced therapeutic potential in resolving Klebsiella pneumoniae mediated burn wound infections. Burns 2017; 43(7): 1532-43. [http://dx.doi.org/10.1016/j.burns.2017.03.029] [PMID: 28502784]

[67]	Chadha P, Katare OP, Chhibber S. *In vivo* efficacy of single phage *versus* phage cocktail in resolving burn wound infection in BALB/c mice. Microb Pathog 2016; 99: 68-77. [http://dx.doi.org/10.1016/j.micpath.2016.08.001] [PMID: 27498362]

[68]	Forti F, Roach DR, Cafora M, *et al.* Design of a broad-range bacteriophage cocktail that reduces

pseudomonas aeruginosa biofilms and treats acute infections in two animal models. Antimicrob Agents Chemother 2018; 62(6): e02573-17.
[http://dx.doi.org/10.1128/AAC.02573-17] [PMID: 29555626]

[69]   Manohar P, Nachimuthu R, Lopes BS. The therapeutic potential of bacteriophages targeting gram-negative bacteria using Galleria mellonella infection model. BMC Microbiol 2018; 18(1): 97.
[http://dx.doi.org/10.1186/s12866-018-1234-4] [PMID: 30170558]

[70]   Chhibber S, Shukla A, Kaur S. Transfersomal phage cocktail is an effective treatment against methicillin-resistant staphylococcus aureus-mediated skin and soft tissue infections. Antimicrob Agents Chemother 2017; 61(10): e02146-16.
[http://dx.doi.org/10.1128/AAC.02146-16] [PMID: 28739792]

[71]   Morris JL, Letson HL, Elliott L, *et al.* Evaluation of bacteriophage as an adjunct therapy for treatment of peri-prosthetic joint infection caused by Staphylococcus aureus. PLoS One 2019; 14(12): e0226574.
[http://dx.doi.org/10.1371/journal.pone.0226574] [PMID: 31877146]

[72]   Geng H, Zou W, Zhang M, *et al.* Evaluation of phage therapy in the treatment of Staphylococcus aureus-induced mastitis in mice. Folia Microbiol (Praha) 2020; 65(2): 339-51.
[http://dx.doi.org/10.1007/s12223-019-00729-9] [PMID: 31256341]

[73]   Torres-Barceló C, Hochberg ME. Evolutionary rationale for phages as complements of antibiotics. Trends Microbiol 2016; 24(4): 249-56.
[http://dx.doi.org/10.1016/j.tim.2015.12.011] [PMID: 26786863]

[74]   Verma V, Harjai K, Chhibber S. Restricting ciprofloxacin-induced resistant variant formation in biofilm of Klebsiella pneumoniae B5055 by complementary bacteriophage treatment. J Antimicrob Chemother 2009; 64(6): 1212-8.
[http://dx.doi.org/10.1093/jac/dkp360] [PMID: 19808232]

[75]   Kirby AE. Synergistic action of gentamicin and bacteriophage in a continuous culture population of Staphylococcus aureus. PLoS One 2012; 7(11): e51017.
[http://dx.doi.org/10.1371/journal.pone.0051017] [PMID: 23226451]

[76]   Torres-Barceló C, Arias-Sánchez FI, Vasse M, Ramsayer J, Kaltz O, Hochberg ME. A window of opportunity to control the bacterial pathogen Pseudomonas aeruginosa combining antibiotics and phages. PLoS One 2014; 9(9): e106628.
[http://dx.doi.org/10.1371/journal.pone.0106628] [PMID: 25259735]

[77]   Kamal F, Dennis JJ. Burkholderia cepacia complex Phage-Antibiotic Synergy (PAS): antibiotics stimulate lytic phage activity. Appl Environ Microbiol 2015; 81(3): 1132-8.
[http://dx.doi.org/10.1128/AEM.02850-14] [PMID: 25452284]

[78]   Oechslin F, Piccardi P, Mancini S, *et al.* Synergistic interaction between phage therapy and antibiotics clears Pseudomonas Aeruginosa infection in endocarditis and reduces virulence. J Infect Dis 2017; 215(5): 703-12.
[PMID: 28007922]

[79]   Chan BK, Sistrom M, Wertz JE, Kortright KE, Narayan D, Turner PE. Phage selection restores antibiotic sensitivity in MDR Pseudomonas aeruginosa. Sci Rep 2016; 6: 26717.
[http://dx.doi.org/10.1038/srep26717] [PMID: 27225966]

[80]   Segall AM, Roach DR, Strathdee SA. Stronger together? Perspectives on phage-antibiotic synergy in clinical applications of phage therapy. Curr Opin Microbiol 2019; 51: 46-50.
[http://dx.doi.org/10.1016/j.mib.2019.03.005] [PMID: 31226502]

[81]   Kim M, Jo Y, Hwang YJ, *et al.* Phage-antibiotic synergy *via* delayed lysis. Appl Environ Microbiol 2018; 84(22): e02085-18.
[http://dx.doi.org/10.1128/AEM.02085-18] [PMID: 30217844]

[82]   Akturk E, Oliveira H, Santos SB, *et al.* Synergistic action of phage and antibiotics: parameters to enhance the killing efficacy against mono and dual-species biofilms. Antibiotics (Basel) 2019; 8(3):

103.
[http://dx.doi.org/10.3390/antibiotics8030103] [PMID: 31349628]

[83]   Uchiyama J, Shigehisa R, Nasukawa T, *et al.* Piperacillin and ceftazidime produce the strongest synergistic phage-antibiotic effect in Pseudomonas aeruginosa. Arch Virol 2018; 163(7): 1941-8.
[http://dx.doi.org/10.1007/s00705-018-3811-0] [PMID: 29550930]

[84]   Kebriaei R, Lev K, Morrisette T, *et al.* Bacteriophage-antibiotic combination strategy: an alternative against methicillin-resistant phenotypes of staphylococcus aureus. Antimicrob Agents Chemother 2020; 64(7): e00461-20.
[http://dx.doi.org/10.1128/AAC.00461-20] [PMID: 32393490]

[85]   Huh H, Wong S, St Jean J, Slavcev R. Bacteriophage interactions with mammalian tissue: Therapeutic applications. Adv Drug Deliv Rev 2019; 145: 4-17.
[http://dx.doi.org/10.1016/j.addr.2019.01.003] [PMID: 30659855]

[86]   Hodyra-Stefaniak K, Miernikiewicz P, Drapała J, *et al.* Mammalian Host-*versus*-Phage immune response determines phage fate *in vivo.* Sci Rep 2015; 5: 14802.
[http://dx.doi.org/10.1038/srep14802] [PMID: 26440922]

[87]   Kakasis A, Panitsa G. Bacteriophage therapy as an alternative treatment for human infections. A comprehensive review. Int J Antimicrob Agents 2019; 53(1): 16-21.
[http://dx.doi.org/10.1016/j.ijantimicag.2018.09.004] [PMID: 30236954]

[88]   Wagner PL, Waldor MK. Bacteriophage control of bacterial virulence. Infect Immun 2002; 70(8): 3985-93.
[http://dx.doi.org/10.1128/IAI.70.8.3985-3993.2002] [PMID: 12117903]

[89]   Garretto A, Miller-Ensminger T, Wolfe AJ, Putonti C. Bacteriophages of the lower urinary tract. Nat Rev Urol 2019; 16(7): 422-32.
[http://dx.doi.org/10.1038/s41585-019-0192-4] [PMID: 31073244]

[90]   Łusiak-Szelachowska M, Weber-Dąbrowska B, Jończyk-Matysiak E, Wojciechowska R, Górski A. Bacteriophages in the gastrointestinal tract and their implications. Gut Pathog 2017; 9: 44.
[http://dx.doi.org/10.1186/s13099-017-0196-7] [PMID: 28811841]

[91]   Van Belleghem JD, Dąbrowska K, Vaneechoutte M, Barr JJ, Bollyky PL. Interactions between bacteriophage, bacteria, and the mammalian immune system. Viruses 2018; 11(1): 11.
[http://dx.doi.org/10.3390/v11010010] [PMID: 30585199]

[92]   Morrison DC, Ulevitch RJ. The effects of bacterial endotoxins on host mediation systems. A review. Am J Pathol 1978; 93(2): 526-618.
[PMID: 362943]

[93]   Cani PD. Human gut microbiome: hopes, threats and promises. Gut 2018; 67(9): 1716-25.
[http://dx.doi.org/10.1136/gutjnl-2018-316723] [PMID: 29934437]

[94]   Carroll-Portillo A, Lin HC. Bacteriophage and the innate immune system: Access and signaling. Microorganisms 2019; 7(12): 7.
[http://dx.doi.org/10.3390/microorganisms7120625] [PMID: 31795262]

[95]   Nguyen S, Baker K, Padman BS, *et al.* Bacteriophage transcytosis provides a mechanism to cross epithelial cell layers. MBio 2017; 8(6): 8.
[http://dx.doi.org/10.1128/mBio.01874-17] [PMID: 29162715]

[96]   Zaczek M, Górski A, Skaradzińska A, Łusiak-Szelachowska M, Weber-D'browska B. Phage penetration of eukaryotic cells: Practical implications. Future Virol 2019; 14: 745-60.
[http://dx.doi.org/10.2217/fvl-2019-0110]

[97]   WaÅna E, DÄ browska B-W, DÄ browska K, ÅwitaÅ a-JeleÅ K, MiÄdzybrodzki R. Bacteriophage translocation. FEMS Immunol Med Microbiol 2006; 46: 313-9.

[98]   Sinha A, Maurice CF. 2019.

[99] Tuma P, Hubbard AL. Transcytosis: crossing cellular barriers. Physiol Rev 2003; 83(3): 871-932.
[http://dx.doi.org/10.1152/physrev.00001.2003] [PMID: 12843411]

[100] Górski A, Dąbrowska K, Międzybrodzki R, *et al.* Phages and immunomodulation. Future Microbiol 2017; 12: 905-14.
[http://dx.doi.org/10.2217/fmb-2017-0049] [PMID: 28434234]

[101] Górski A, Międzybrodzki R, Borysowski J, *et al.* Phage as a modulator of immune responses: practical implications for phage therapy. Adv Virus Res 2012; 83: 41-71.
[http://dx.doi.org/10.1016/B978-0-12-394438-2.00002-5] [PMID: 22748808]

[102] Żaczek M, Łusiak-Szelachowska M, Weber-Dąbrowska B, *et al.* Humoral immune response to phage-based therapeutics. Phage Ther. A Pract. Approach 2019; pp. 123-43.

[103] Jariah ROA, Hakim MS. Interaction of phages, bacteria, and the human immune system: Evolutionary changes in phage therapy. Rev Med Virol 2019; 29(5): e2055.
[http://dx.doi.org/10.1002/rmv.2055] [PMID: 31145517]

[104] Dabrowska K, Switała-Jelen K, Opolski A, Weber-Dabrowska B, Gorski A. Bacteriophage penetration in vertebrates. J Appl Microbiol 2005; 98(1): 7-13.
[http://dx.doi.org/10.1111/j.1365-2672.2004.02422.x] [PMID: 15610412]

[105] Borysowski J, Górski A. Is phage therapy acceptable in the immunocompromised host? Int J Infect Dis 2008; 12(5): 466-71.
[http://dx.doi.org/10.1016/j.ijid.2008.01.006] [PMID: 18400541]

[106] Górski A, Jończyk-Matysiak E, Łusiak-Szelachowska M, Międzybrodzki R, Weber-Dąbrowska B, Borysowski J. Phage therapy in allergic disorders? Exp Biol Med (Maywood) 2018; 243(6): 534-7.
[http://dx.doi.org/10.1177/1535370218755658] [PMID: 29359577]

[107] Lack G, Ochs HD, Gelfand EW. Humoral immunity in steroid-dependent children with asthma and hypogammaglobulinemia. J Pediatr 1996; 129(6): 898-903.
[http://dx.doi.org/10.1016/S0022-3476(96)70035-5] [PMID: 8969733]

[108] Krut O, Bekeredjian-Ding I. Contribution of the Immune Response to Phage Therapy. J Immunol 2018; 200(9): 3037-44.
[http://dx.doi.org/10.4049/jimmunol.1701745] [PMID: 29685950]

[109] Fluckiger A, Daillère R, Sassi M, Sixt BS, Liu P, Loos F, *et al.* 2020.

[110] Kucharewicz-Krukowska A, Slopek S. Immunogenic effect of bacteriophage in patients subjected to phage therapy. Arch Immunol Ther Exp (Warsz) 1987; 35(5): 553-61.
[PMID: 3455646]

[111] Bruttin A, Brüssow H. Human volunteers receiving *Escherichia coli* phage T4 orally: a safety test of phage therapy. Antimicrob Agents Chemother 2005; 49(7): 2874-8.
[http://dx.doi.org/10.1128/AAC.49.7.2874-2878.2005] [PMID: 15980363]

[112] 2014.

[113] Malik DJ, Sokolov IJ, Vinner GK, *et al.* Formulation, stabilisation and encapsulation of bacteriophage for phage therapy. Adv Colloid Interface Sci 2017; 249: 100-33.
[http://dx.doi.org/10.1016/j.cis.2017.05.014] [PMID: 28688779]

[114] Górski A, Międzybrodzki R, Łobocka M, *et al.* Phage therapy: What have we learned? Viruses 2018; 10(6): 10.
[http://dx.doi.org/10.3390/v10060288] [PMID: 29843391]

[115] Kurzępa A, Dąbrowska K, Skaradziński G, Górski A. Bacteriophage interactions with phagocytes and their potential significance in experimental therapy. Clin Exp Med 2009; 9(2): 93-100.
[http://dx.doi.org/10.1007/s10238-008-0027-8] [PMID: 19184327]

[116] Roach DR, Leung CY, Henry M, *et al.* Synergy between the host immune system and bacteriophage is

essential for successful phage therapy against an acute respiratory pathogen. Cell Host Microbe 2017; 22(1): 38-47.e4.
[http://dx.doi.org/10.1016/j.chom.2017.06.018] [PMID: 28704651]

[117]   Żaczek M, Łusiak-Szelachowska M, Jończyk-Matysiak E, *et al.* Antibody production in response to staphylococcal MS-1 phage cocktail in patients undergoing phage therapy. Front Microbiol 2016; 7: 1681.
[http://dx.doi.org/10.3389/fmicb.2016.01681] [PMID: 27822205]

[118]   Leung CYJ, Weitz JS. Modeling the synergistic elimination of bacteria by phage and the innate immune system. J Theor Biol 2017; 429: 241-52.
[http://dx.doi.org/10.1016/j.jtbi.2017.06.037] [PMID: 28668337]

[119]   Abedon ST. Phage therapy: eco-physiological pharmacology. Scientifica (Cairo) 2014; 2014: 581639.
[http://dx.doi.org/10.1155/2014/581639] [PMID: 25031881]

[120]   Dąbrowska K. Phage therapy: What factors shape phage pharmacokinetics and bioavailability? Systematic and critical review. Med Res Rev 2019; 39(5): 2000-25.
[http://dx.doi.org/10.1002/med.21572] [PMID: 30887551]

[121]   Manohar P, Tamhankar AJ, Leptihn S, Ramesh N. Pharmacological and Immunological Aspects of Phage Therapy. Infect Microbes Dis 2019; 1: 34-42.
[http://dx.doi.org/10.1097/IM9.0000000000000013]

[122]   Bull JJ, Regoes RR. Pharmacodynamics of non-replicating viruses, bacteriocins and lysins. Proc Biol Sci 2006; 273(1602): 2703-12.
[http://dx.doi.org/10.1098/rspb.2006.3640] [PMID: 17015317]

[123]   Nilsson AS. Pharmacological limitations of phage therapy. Ups J Med Sci 2019; 124(4): 218-27.
[http://dx.doi.org/10.1080/03009734.2019.1688433] [PMID: 31724901]

[124]   Abedon S. Phage therapy pharmacology: calculating phage dosing. Adv Appl Microbiol 2011; 77: 1-40.
[http://dx.doi.org/10.1016/B978-0-12-387044-5.00001-7] [PMID: 22050820]

[125]   Qadir MI, Mobeen T, Masood A. Phage therapy: Progress in pharmacokinetics. Braz J Pharm Sci 2018; 54: 17093.
[http://dx.doi.org/10.1590/s2175-97902018000117093]

[126]   Dąbrowska K, Abedon ST. Pharmacologically aware phage therapy: pharmacodynamic and pharmacokinetic obstacles to phage antibacterial action in animal and human bodies. Microbiol Mol Biol Rev 2019; 83(4): 83.
[http://dx.doi.org/10.1128/MMBR.00012-19] [PMID: 31666296]

[127]   Ross A, Ward S, Hyman P. More is better: selecting for broad host range bacteriophages. Front Microbiol 2016; 7: 1352.
[http://dx.doi.org/10.3389/fmicb.2016.01352] [PMID: 27660623]

[128]   Ramesh N, Archana L, Madurantakam Royam M, Manohar P, Eniyan K. Effect of various bacteriological media on the plaque morphology of *Staphylococcus* and *Vibrio* phages. Access Microbiol 2019; 1(4): e000036.
[http://dx.doi.org/10.1099/acmi.0.000036] [PMID: 32974524]

[129]   Gadagkar R, Gopinathan KP. Bacteriophage burst size during multiple infections. J Biosci 1980; 2: 253-9.
[http://dx.doi.org/10.1007/BF02703251]

[130]   Choińska-Pulit A, Mituła P, Śliwka P, Łaba W, Skaradzińska A. Bacteriophage encapsulation: Trends and potential applications. Trends Food Sci Technol 2015; 45: 212-21.
[http://dx.doi.org/10.1016/j.tifs.2015.07.001]

[131]   Abdelsattar AS, Abdelrahman F, Dawoud A, Connerton IF, El-Shibiny A. Encapsulation of E. coli phage ZCEC5 in chitosan-alginate beads as a delivery system in phage therapy. AMB Express 2019;

9(1): 87.
[http://dx.doi.org/10.1186/s13568-019-0810-9] [PMID: 31209685]

[132]  Abedon S. Phage Therapy Pharmacology 2011.
[http://dx.doi.org/10.1016/B978-0-12-387044-5.00001-7]

[133]  Moldovan R, Chapman-McQuiston E, Wu XL. On kinetics of phage adsorption. Biophys J 2007; 93(1): 303-15.
[http://dx.doi.org/10.1529/biophysj.106.102962] [PMID: 17434950]

[134]  Ryan EM, Gorman SP, Donnelly RF, Gilmore BF. Recent advances in bacteriophage therapy: how delivery routes, formulation, concentration and timing influence the success of phage therapy. J Pharm Pharmacol 2011; 63(10): 1253-64.
[http://dx.doi.org/10.1111/j.2042-7158.2011.01324.x] [PMID: 21899540]

[135]  Chang RYK, Wallin M, Lin Y, *et al.* Phage therapy for respiratory infections. Adv Drug Deliv Rev 2018; 133: 76-86.
[http://dx.doi.org/10.1016/j.addr.2018.08.001] [PMID: 30096336]

[136]  Tiwari BR, Kim S, Rahman M, Kim J. Antibacterial efficacy of lytic Pseudomonas bacteriophage in normal and neutropenic mice models. J Microbiol 2011; 49(6): 994-9.
[http://dx.doi.org/10.1007/s12275-011-1512-4] [PMID: 22203564]

[137]  Wroe JA, Johnson CT, García AJ. Bacteriophage delivering hydrogels reduce biofilm formation *in vitro* and infection *in vivo.* J Biomed Mater Res A 2020; 108(1): 39-49.
[http://dx.doi.org/10.1002/jbm.a.36790] [PMID: 31443115]

[138]  Najar MS, Saldanha CL, Banday KA. Approach to urinary tract infections. Indian J Nephrol 2009; 19(4): 129-39.
[http://dx.doi.org/10.4103/0971-4065.59333] [PMID: 20535247]

[139]  Inchley CJ. The actvity of mouse Kupffer cells following intravenous injection of T4 bacteriophage. Clin Exp Immunol 1969; 5(1): 173-87.
[PMID: 5370053]

[140]  Hooper L V. Commensal Host-Bacterial Relationships in the Gut 2001.
[http://dx.doi.org/10.1126/science.1058709]

[141]  Grice EA, Segre JA. The skin microbiome. Nat Rev Microbiol 2011; 9(4): 244-53.
[http://dx.doi.org/10.1038/nrmicro2537] [PMID: 21407241]

[142]  Church D, Elsayed S, Reid O, Winston B, Lindsay R. Burn wound infections. Clin Microbiol Rev 2006; 19(2): 403-34.
[http://dx.doi.org/10.1128/CMR.19.2.403-434.2006] [PMID: 16614255]

[143]  Rafla K, Tredget EE. Infection control in the burn unit. Burns 2011; 37(1): 5-15.
[http://dx.doi.org/10.1016/j.burns.2009.06.198] [PMID: 20561750]

[144]  Shera G. Phage treatment of severe burns. BMJ 1970; 1(5695): 568-9.
[http://dx.doi.org/10.1136/bmj.1.5695.568-b] [PMID: 5435214]

[145]  McVay CS, Velásquez M, Fralick JA. Phage therapy of Pseudomonas aeruginosa infection in a mouse burn wound model. Antimicrob Agents Chemother 2007; 51(6): 1934-8.
[http://dx.doi.org/10.1128/AAC.01028-06] [PMID: 17387151]

[146]  Merabishvili M, Pirnay J-P, Verbeken G, *et al.* Quality-controlled small-scale production of a well-defined bacteriophage cocktail for use in human clinical trials. PLoS One 2009; 4(3): e4944.
[http://dx.doi.org/10.1371/journal.pone.0004944] [PMID: 19300511]

[147]  Malik R, Chhibber S. Protection with bacteriophage KØ1 against fatal Klebsiella pneumoniae-induced burn wound infection in mice. J Microbiol Immunol Infect 2009; 42(2): 134-40.
[PMID: 19597645]

[148]  Kumari S, Harjai K, Chhibber S. Efficacy of bacteriophage treatment in murine burn wound infection

induced by klebsiella pneumoniae. J Microbiol Biotechnol 2009; 19(6): 622-8.
[http://dx.doi.org/10.4014/jmb.0808.493] [PMID: 19597322]

[149] Kumari S, Harjai K, Chhibber S. Bacteriophage *versus* antimicrobial agents for the treatment of murine burn wound infection caused by Klebsiella pneumoniae B5055. J Med Microbiol 2011; 60(Pt 2): 205-10.
[http://dx.doi.org/10.1099/jmm.0.018580-0] [PMID: 20965914]

[150] Meurice E, Rguiti E, Brutel A, *et al.* New antibacterial microporous CaP materials loaded with phages for prophylactic treatment in bone surgery. J Mater Sci Mater Med 2012; 23(10): 2445-52.
[http://dx.doi.org/10.1007/s10856-012-4711-6] [PMID: 22802104]

[151] Chhibber S, Kaur T, Sandeep Kaur . Co-therapy using lytic bacteriophage and linezolid: effective treatment in eliminating methicillin resistant Staphylococcus aureus (MRSA) from diabetic foot infections. PLoS One 2013; 8(2): e56022.
[http://dx.doi.org/10.1371/journal.pone.0056022] [PMID: 23418497]

[152] Mendes JJ, Leandro C, Corte-Real S, *et al.* Wound healing potential of topical bacteriophage therapy on diabetic cutaneous wounds. Wound Repair Regen 2013; 21(4): 595-603.
[http://dx.doi.org/10.1111/wrr.12056] [PMID: 23755910]

[153] Shivaswamy VC, Kalasuramath SB, Sadanand CK, *et al.* Ability of bacteriophage in resolving wound infection caused by multidrug-resistant Acinetobacter baumannii in uncontrolled diabetic rats. Microb Drug Resist 2015; 21(2): 171-7.
[http://dx.doi.org/10.1089/mdr.2014.0120] [PMID: 25411824]

[154] Basu S, Agarwal M, Kumar Bhartiya S, Nath G, Kumar Shukla V. An *in vivo* Wound Model Utilizing Bacteriophage Therapy of Pseudomonas aeruginosa Biofilms. Ostomy Wound Manage 2015; 61(8): 16-23.
[PMID: 26291897]

[155] Chhibber S, Kaur J, Kaur S. Liposome entrapment of bacteriophages improves wound healing in a diabetic mouse mrsa infection. Front Microbiol 2018; 9: 561.
[http://dx.doi.org/10.3389/fmicb.2018.00561] [PMID: 29651276]

[156] Oliveira A, Sousa JC, Silva AC, Melo LDR, Sillankorva S. Chestnut honey and bacteriophage application to control *pseudomonas aeruginosa and escherichia coli* biofilms: evaluation in an *ex vivo* wound model. Front Microbiol 2018; 9: 1725.
[http://dx.doi.org/10.3389/fmicb.2018.01725] [PMID: 30108574]

[157] Gupta P, Singh HS, Shukla VK, Nath G, Bhartiya SK. Bacteriophage therapy of chronic nonhealing wound: clinical study. Int J Low Extrem Wounds 2019; 18(2): 171-5.
[http://dx.doi.org/10.1177/1534734619835115] [PMID: 31081402]

[158] Sarhan WA, Azzazy HM. Apitherapeutics and phage-loaded nanofibers as wound dressings with enhanced wound healing and antibacterial activity. Nanomedicine (Lond) 2017; 12(17): 2055-67.
[http://dx.doi.org/10.2217/nnm-2017-0151] [PMID: 28805554]

[159] Kaur P, Gondil VS, Chhibber S. A novel wound dressing consisting of PVA-SA hybrid hydrogel membrane for topical delivery of bacteriophages and antibiotics. Int J Pharm 2019; 572: 118779.
[http://dx.doi.org/10.1016/j.ijpharm.2019.118779] [PMID: 31740093]

[160] Kifelew LG, Warner MS, Morales S, *et al.* Efficacy of phage cocktail AB-SA01 therapy in diabetic mouse wound infections caused by multidrug-resistant Staphylococcus aureus. BMC Microbiol 2020; 20(1): 204.
[http://dx.doi.org/10.1186/s12866-020-01891-8] [PMID: 32646376]

[161] Rubio TT. Infection in patients with cystic fibrosis. Am J Med 1986; 81(1A): 73-7.
[http://dx.doi.org/10.1016/0002-9343(86)90516-4] [PMID: 3526881]

[162] Jones RN. Microbial etiologies of hospital-acquired bacterial pneumonia and ventilator-associated bacterial pneumonia. Clin Infect Dis 2010; 51 (Suppl. 1): S81-7.

[http://dx.doi.org/10.1086/653053] [PMID: 20597676]

[163] Gómez MI, Prince A. Opportunistic infections in lung disease: Pseudomonas infections in cystic fibrosis. Curr Opin Pharmacol 2007; 7(3): 244-51.
[http://dx.doi.org/10.1016/j.coph.2006.12.005] [PMID: 17418640]

[164] Criscuolo E, Spadini S, Lamanna J, Ferro M, Burioni R. Bacteriophages and Their Immunological Applications against Infectious Threats. J Immunol Res 2017; 2017: 3780697.
[http://dx.doi.org/10.1155/2017/3780697] [PMID: 28484722]

[165] Debarbieux L, Leduc D, Maura D, et al. Bacteriophages can treat and prevent Pseudomonas aeruginosa lung infections. J Infect Dis 2010; 201(7): 1096-104.
[http://dx.doi.org/10.1086/651135] [PMID: 20196657]

[166] Morello E, Saussereau E, Maura D, Huerre M, Touqui L, Debarbieux L. Pulmonary bacteriophage therapy on Pseudomonas aeruginosa cystic fibrosis strains: first steps towards treatment and prevention. PLoS One 2011; 6(2): e16963.
[http://dx.doi.org/10.1371/journal.pone.0016963] [PMID: 21347240]

[167] Seed KD, Dennis JJ. Experimental bacteriophage therapy increases survival of Galleria mellonella larvae infected with clinically relevant strains of the Burkholderia cepacia complex. Antimicrob Agents Chemother 2009; 53(5): 2205-8.
[http://dx.doi.org/10.1128/AAC.01166-08] [PMID: 19223640]

[168] Carmody LA, Gill JJ, Summer EJ, et al. Efficacy of bacteriophage therapy in a model of Burkholderia cenocepacia pulmonary infection. J Infect Dis 2010; 201(2): 264-71.
[http://dx.doi.org/10.1086/649227] [PMID: 20001604]

[169] Alemayehu D, Casey PG, McAuliffe O, et al. Bacteriophages φMR299-2 and φNH-4 can eliminate Pseudomonas aeruginosa in the murine lung and on cystic fibrosis lung airway cells. MBio 2012; 3(2): e00029-12.
[http://dx.doi.org/10.1128/mBio.00029-12] [PMID: 22396480]

[170] Lynch KH, Liang Y, Eberl L, Wishart DS, Dennis JJ. Identification and characterization of φH111-1: A novel myovirus with broad activity against clinical isolates of *Burkholderia cenocepacia*. Bacteriophage 2013; 3(4): e26649.
[http://dx.doi.org/10.4161/bact.26649] [PMID: 24265978]

[171] Sahota JS, Smith CM, Radhakrishnan P, et al. Bacteriophage Delivery by Nebulization and Efficacy Against Phenotypically Diverse Pseudomonas aeruginosa from Cystic Fibrosis Patients. J Aerosol Med Pulm Drug Deliv 2015; 28(5): 353-60.
[http://dx.doi.org/10.1089/jamp.2014.1172] [PMID: 25714328]

[172] Olszak T, Zarnowiec P, Kaca W, et al. In vitro and in vivo antibacterial activity of environmental bacteriophages against Pseudomonas aeruginosa strains from cystic fibrosis patients. Appl Microbiol Biotechnol 2015; 99(14): 6021-33.
[http://dx.doi.org/10.1007/s00253-015-6492-6] [PMID: 25758956]

[173] Pabary R, Singh C, Morales S, et al. Antipseudomonal Bacteriophage Reduces Infective Burden and Inflammatory Response in Murine Lung. Antimicrob Agents Chemother 2015; 60(2): 744-51.
[http://dx.doi.org/10.1128/AAC.01426-15] [PMID: 26574007]

[174] Waters EM, Neill DR, Kaman B, et al. Phage therapy is highly effective against chronic lung infections with *Pseudomonas aeruginosa*. Thorax 2017; 72(7): 666-7.
[http://dx.doi.org/10.1136/thoraxjnl-2016-209265] [PMID: 28265031]

[175] Shiley JR, Comfort KK, Robinson JB. Immunogenicity and antimicrobial effectiveness of Pseudomonas aeruginosa specific bacteriophage in a human lung *in vitro* model. Appl Microbiol Biotechnol 2017; 101(21): 7977-85.
[http://dx.doi.org/10.1007/s00253-017-8504-1] [PMID: 28914348]

[176] Lin Y, Chang RYK, Britton WJ, Morales S, Kutter E, Chan H-K. Synergy of nebulized phage PEV20

and ciprofloxacin combination against Pseudomonas aeruginosa. Int J Pharm 2018; 551(1-2): 158-65. [http://dx.doi.org/10.1016/j.ijpharm.2018.09.024] [PMID: 30223075]

[177]    Hoyle N, Zhvaniya P, Balarjishvili N, *et al.* Phage therapy against Achromobacter xylosoxidans lung infection in a patient with cystic fibrosis: a case report. Res Microbiol 2018; 169(9): 540-2. [http://dx.doi.org/10.1016/j.resmic.2018.05.001] [PMID: 29777836]

[178]    Cafora M, Deflorian G, Forti F, *et al.* Phage therapy against Pseudomonas aeruginosa infections in a cystic fibrosis zebrafish model. Sci Rep 2019; 9(1): 1527. [http://dx.doi.org/10.1038/s41598-018-37636-x] [PMID: 30728389]

[179]    Law N, Logan C, Yung G, *et al.* Successful adjunctive use of bacteriophage therapy for treatment of multidrug-resistant Pseudomonas aeruginosa infection in a cystic fibrosis patient. Infection 2019; 47(4): 665-8. [http://dx.doi.org/10.1007/s15010-019-01319-0] [PMID: 31102236]

[180]    Gainey AB, Burch A, Brownstein MJ, *et al.* Combining bacteriophages with cefiderocol and meropenem/vaborbactam to treat a pan-drug resistant Achromobacter species infection in a pediatric cystic fibrosis patient. Pediatr Pulmonol 2020; 55: 2990-4.

[181]    Foxman B. Urinary tract infection syndromes: occurrence, recurrence, bacteriology, risk factors, and disease burden. Infect Dis Clin North Am 2014; 28(1): 1-13. [http://dx.doi.org/10.1016/j.idc.2013.09.003] [PMID: 24484571]

[182]    Flores-Mireles AL, Walker JN, Caparon M, Hultgren SJ. Urinary tract infections: epidemiology, mechanisms of infection and treatment options. Nat Rev Microbiol 2015; 13(5): 269-84. [http://dx.doi.org/10.1038/nrmicro3432] [PMID: 25853778]

[183]    Malik S, Sidhu PK, Rana JS, Nehra K. Managing urinary tract infections through phage therapy: a novel approach. Folia Microbiol (Praha) 2020; 65(2): 217-31. [http://dx.doi.org/10.1007/s12223-019-00750-y] [PMID: 31494814]

[184]    Zalewska-Piątek B, Piątek R. Phage Therapy as a Novel Strategy in the Treatment of Urinary Tract Infections Caused by *E. Coli.* Antibiotics (Basel) 2020; 9(6): 304. [http://dx.doi.org/10.3390/antibiotics9060304] [PMID: 32517088]

[185]    Zalewska-Piątek B, Piątek R, Krawczyk B, Olszewski M. Pathomechanism of urinary tract infections caused by uropathogenic E. coli strains. Postepy Hig Med Dosw 2019; 73: 269-81. [http://dx.doi.org/10.5604/01.3001.0013.2022]

[186]    Ujmajuridze A, Chanishvili N, Goderdzishvili M, *et al.* Adapted bacteriophages for treating urinary tract infections. Front Microbiol 2018; 9: 1832. [http://dx.doi.org/10.3389/fmicb.2018.01832] [PMID: 30131795]

[187]    Nishikawa H, Yasuda M, Uchiyama J, *et al.* T-even-related bacteriophages as candidates for treatment of *Escherichia coli* urinary tract infections. Arch Virol 2008; 153(3): 507-15. [http://dx.doi.org/10.1007/s00705-007-0031-4] [PMID: 18188500]

[188]    Sillankorva S, Oliveira D, Moura A, *et al.* Efficacy of a broad host range lytic bacteriophage against E. coli adhered to urothelium. Curr Microbiol 2011; 62(4): 1128-32. [http://dx.doi.org/10.1007/s00284-010-9834-8] [PMID: 21140149]

[189]    Tóthová L, Celec P, Bábíčková J, *et al.* Phage therapy of Cronobacter-induced urinary tract infection in mice 2011. [http://dx.doi.org/10.12659/MSM.881844]

[190]    Chibeu A, Lingohr EJ, Masson L, *et al.* Bacteriophages with the ability to degrade uropathogenic *Escherichia coli* biofilms. Viruses 2012; 4(4): 471-87. [http://dx.doi.org/10.3390/v4040471] [PMID: 22590682]

[191]    Nzakizwanayo J, Hanin A, Alves DR, *et al.* Bacteriophage can prevent encrustation and blockage of urinary catheters by proteus mirabilis. Antimicrob Agents Chemother 2015; 60(3): 1530-6. [http://dx.doi.org/10.1128/AAC.02685-15] [PMID: 26711744]

[192] Melo LDR, Veiga P, Cerca N, *et al.* Development of a phage cocktail to control proteus mirabilis catheter-associated urinary tract infections. Front Microbiol 2016; 7: 1024.
[http://dx.doi.org/10.3389/fmicb.2016.01024] [PMID: 27446059]

[193] Leitner L, Sybesma W, Chanishvili N, *et al.* Bacteriophages for treating urinary tract infections in patients undergoing transurethral resection of the prostate: a randomized, placebo-controlled, double-blind clinical trial. BMC Urol 2017; 17(1): 90.
[http://dx.doi.org/10.1186/s12894-017-0283-6] [PMID: 28950849]

[194] Yazdi M, Bouzari M, Ghaemi EA. Isolation and characterization of a lytic bacteriophage (vb_pmis-th) and its application in combination with ampicillin against planktonic and biofilm forms of proteus mirabilis isolated from urinary tract infection. J Mol Microbiol Biotechnol 2018; 28(1): 37-46.
[http://dx.doi.org/10.1159/000487137] [PMID: 29617701]

[195] Gu Y, Xu Y, Xu J, *et al.* Identification of novel bacteriophage vB_EcoP-EG1 with lytic activity against planktonic and biofilm forms of uropathogenic *Escherichia coli.* Appl Microbiol Biotechnol 2019; 103(1): 315-26.
[http://dx.doi.org/10.1007/s00253-018-9471-x] [PMID: 30397766]

[196] Moradpour Z, Yousefi N, Sadeghi D, Ghasemian A. Synergistic bactericidal activity of a naturally isolated phage and ampicillin against urinary tract infecting *Escherichia coli* O157. Iran J Basic Med Sci 2020; 23(2): 257-63.
[http://dx.doi.org/10.22038/IJBMS.2019.37561.8989] [PMID: 32405370]

[197] Grygorcewicz B, Wojciuk B, Roszak M, *et al.* Environmental phage-based cocktail and antibiotic combination effects on acinetobacter baumannii biofilm in a human urine model 2020.
[http://dx.doi.org/10.1089/mdr.2020.0083]

[198] Rostkowska OM, Międzybrodzki R, Miszewska□Szyszkowska D, Górski A, Durlik M. Treatment of recurrent urinary tract infections in a 60-year-old kidney transplant recipient. The use of phage therapy. Transpl Infect Dis 2021; 23(1): e13391.

[199] Hoe S, Semler DD, Goudie AD, *et al.* Respirable bacteriophages for the treatment of bacterial lung infections. J Aerosol Med Pulm Drug Deliv 2013; 26(6): 317-35.
[http://dx.doi.org/10.1089/jamp.2012.1001] [PMID: 23597003]

[200] Abedon ST. Phage therapy of pulmonary infections. Bacteriophage 2015; 5(1): e1020260.
[http://dx.doi.org/10.1080/21597081.2015.1020260] [PMID: 26442188]

[201] Chhibber S, Kaur S, Kumari S. Therapeutic potential of bacteriophage in treating Klebsiella pneumoniae B5055-mediated lobar pneumonia in mice. J Med Microbiol 2008; 57(Pt 12): 1508-13.
[http://dx.doi.org/10.1099/jmm.0.2008/002873-0] [PMID: 19018021]

[202] Shen G-H, Wang J-L, Wen F-S, *et al.* Isolation and characterization of φkm18p, a novel lytic phage with therapeutic potential against extensively drug resistant Acinetobacter baumannii. PLoS One 2012; 7(10): e46537.
[http://dx.doi.org/10.1371/journal.pone.0046537] [PMID: 23071586]

[203] Drilling A, Morales S, Jardeleza C, Vreugde S, Speck P, Wormald P-J. Bacteriophage reduces biofilm of Staphylococcus aureus *ex vivo* isolates from chronic rhinosinusitis patients. Am J Rhinol Allergy 2014; 28(1): 3-11.
[http://dx.doi.org/10.2500/ajra.2014.28.4001] [PMID: 24717868]

[204] Takemura-Uchiyama I, Uchiyama J, Osanai M, *et al.* Experimental phage therapy against lethal lung-derived septicemia caused by Staphylococcus aureus in mice. Microbes Infect 2014; 16(6): 512-7.
[http://dx.doi.org/10.1016/j.micinf.2014.02.011] [PMID: 24631574]

[205] Singla S, Harjai K, Katare OP, Chhibber S. Bacteriophage-loaded nanostructured lipid carrier: improved pharmacokinetics mediates effective resolution of Klebsiella pneumoniae-induced lobar pneumonia. J Infect Dis 2015; 212(2): 325-34.
[http://dx.doi.org/10.1093/infdis/jiv029] [PMID: 25605867]

[206]  Wang Y, Mi Z, Niu W, *et al.* Intranasal treatment with bacteriophage rescues mice from Acinetobacter baumannii-mediated pneumonia. Future Microbiol 2016; 11: 631-41.
[http://dx.doi.org/10.2217/fmb.16.11] [PMID: 26925593]

[207]  Chang RY, Wong J, Mathai A, *et al.* Production of highly stable spray dried phage formulations for treatment of Pseudomonas aeruginosa lung infection. Eur J Pharm Biopharm 2017; 121: 1-13.
[http://dx.doi.org/10.1016/j.ejpb.2017.09.002] [PMID: 28890220]

[208]  Chang RYK, Chen K, Wang J, *et al.* Proof-of-Principle Study in a Murine Lung Infection Model of Antipseudomonal Activity of Phage PEV20 in a Dry-Powder Formulation. Antimicrob Agents Chemother 2018; 62(2): e01714-17.
[http://dx.doi.org/10.1128/AAC.01714-17] [PMID: 29158280]

[209]  Jeon J, Park J-H, Yong D. Efficacy of bacteriophage treatment against carbapenem-resistant Acinetobacter baumannii in Galleria mellonella larvae and a mouse model of acute pneumonia. BMC Microbiol 2019; 19(1): 70.
[http://dx.doi.org/10.1186/s12866-019-1443-5] [PMID: 30940074]

[210]  Jeon J, Yong D. Two Novel Bacteriophages Improve Survival in *Galleria mellonella* Infection and Mouse Acute Pneumonia Models Infected with Extensively Drug-Resistant *Pseudomonas aeruginosa.* Appl Environ Microbiol 2019; 85(9): e02900-18.
[http://dx.doi.org/10.1128/AEM.02900-18] [PMID: 30824445]

[211]  Prazak J, Iten M, Cameron DR, *et al.* Bacteriophages Improve Outcomes in Experimental *Staphylococcus aureus* Ventilator-associated Pneumonia. Am J Respir Crit Care Med 2019; 200(9): 1126-33.
[http://dx.doi.org/10.1164/rccm.201812-2372OC] [PMID: 31260638]

[212]  Fong SA, Drilling A, Morales S, *et al.* Activity of bacteriophages in removing biofilms of *pseudomonas aeruginosa* isolates from chronic rhinosinusitis patients. Front Cell Infect Microbiol 2017; 7: 418.
[http://dx.doi.org/10.3389/fcimb.2017.00418] [PMID: 29018773]

[213]  Semler DD, Goudie AD, Finlay WH, Dennis JJ. Aerosol phage therapy efficacy in Burkholderia cepacia complex respiratory infections. Antimicrob Agents Chemother 2014; 58(7): 4005-13.
[http://dx.doi.org/10.1128/AAC.02388-13] [PMID: 24798268]

[214]  Kingwell K. Bacteriophage therapies re-enter clinical trials. Nat Rev Drug Discov 2015; 14(8): 515-6.
[http://dx.doi.org/10.1038/nrd4695] [PMID: 26228748]

[215]  Love MJ, Bhandari D, Dobson RCJ, Billington C. Potential for bacteriophage endolysins to supplement or replace antibiotics in food production and clinical care. Antibiotics (Basel) 2018; 7(1): 17.
[http://dx.doi.org/10.3390/antibiotics7010017] [PMID: 29495476]

[216]  Anomaly J. The future of phage: ethical challenges of using phage therapy to treat bacterial infections. Public Health Ethics 2020; 13(1): 82-8.
[http://dx.doi.org/10.1093/phe/phaa003] [PMID: 32760449]

[217]  Pires DP, Costa AR, Pinto G, Meneses L, Azeredo J. Current challenges and future opportunities of phage therapy. FEMS Microbiol Rev 2020; 44(6): 684-700.
[http://dx.doi.org/10.1093/femsre/fuaa017] [PMID: 32472938]

[218]  Oliveira A, Sereno R, Azeredo J. *In vivo* efficiency evaluation of a phage cocktail in controlling severe colibacillosis in confined conditions and experimental poultry houses. Vet Microbiol 2010; 146(3-4): 303-8.
[http://dx.doi.org/10.1016/j.vetmic.2010.05.015] [PMID: 20605377]

[219]  Alves D, Marques A, Milho C, *et al.* Bacteriophage φIBB-PF7A loaded on sodium alginate-based films to prevent microbial meat spoilage. Int J Food Microbiol 2019; 291: 121-7.
[http://dx.doi.org/10.1016/j.ijfoodmicro.2018.11.026] [PMID: 30496941]

[220] Withey S, Cartmell E, Avery LM, Stephenson T. Bacteriophages--potential for application in wastewater treatment processes. Sci Total Environ 2005; 339(1-3): 1-18.
[http://dx.doi.org/10.1016/j.scitotenv.2004.09.021] [PMID: 15740754]

[221] Jassim SAA, Limoges RG, El-Cheikh H. Bacteriophage biocontrol in wastewater treatment. World J Microbiol Biotechnol 2016; 32(4): 70.
[http://dx.doi.org/10.1007/s11274-016-2028-1] [PMID: 26941243]

[222] Shin J, Jardine P, Noireaux V. Genome replication, synthesis, and assembly of the bacteriophage T7 in a single cell-free reaction. ACS Synth Biol 2012; 1(9): 408-13.
[http://dx.doi.org/10.1021/sb300049p] [PMID: 23651338]

[223] Reyes A, Haynes M, Hanson N, *et al.* Viruses in the faecal microbiota of monozygotic twins and their mothers. Nature 2010; 466(7304): 334-8.
[http://dx.doi.org/10.1038/nature09199] [PMID: 20631792]

[224] Amgarten D, Braga LPP, da Silva AM, Setubal JC. MARVEL, a tool for prediction of bacteriophage sequences in metagenomic bins. Front Genet 2018; 9: 304.
[http://dx.doi.org/10.3389/fgene.2018.00304] [PMID: 30131825]

[225] Fernández-Ruiz I, Coutinho FH, Rodriguez-Valera F. Thousands of novel endolysins discovered in uncultured phage genomes. Front Microbiol 2018; 9: 1033.
[http://dx.doi.org/10.3389/fmicb.2018.01033] [PMID: 29867909]

[226] Cahill J, Young R. Phage Lysis: Multiple Genes for Multiple Barriers. Adv Virus Res 2019; 103: 33-70.
[http://dx.doi.org/10.1016/bs.aivir.2018.09.003] [PMID: 30635077]

[227] Schmelcher M, Loessner MJ. Bacteriophage endolysins: applications for food safety. Curr Opin Biotechnol 2016; 37: 76-87.
[http://dx.doi.org/10.1016/j.copbio.2015.10.005] [PMID: 26707470]

[228] Pires DP, Cleto S, Sillankorva S, Azeredo J, Lu TK. Genetically engineered phages: a review of advances over the last decade. Microbiol Mol Biol Rev 2016; 80(3): 523-43.
[http://dx.doi.org/10.1128/MMBR.00069-15] [PMID: 27250768]

[229] Luong T, Salabarria A-C, Edwards RA, Roach DR. Standardized bacteriophage purification for personalized phage therapy. Nat Protoc 2020; 15(9): 2867-90.
[http://dx.doi.org/10.1038/s41596-020-0346-0] [PMID: 32709990]

# CHAPTER 4

# Quorum Sensing Inhibitors from Natural Products: A New Anti-infective Approach

**Debaprasad Parai[1,*], Pia Dey[2]** and **Samir Kumar Mukherjee[2]**

[1] *ICMR-Regional Medical Research Centre, Bhubaneswar, India*

[2] *Department of Microbiology, University of Kalyani, Kalyani, West Bengal, India*

**Abstract:** Currently, the World Health Organization (WHO) considers antibiotic resistance a serious threat to the treatment of infectious diseases. Moreover, the WHO has promoted a complex action plan, based on the slogan "no action today, no cure tomorrow" to control the occurrence and spread of resistant strains that include strategic actions for mitigation, prevention and control. In the last 50 years, only three new classes of antibiotics have been approved by WHO and US Food and Drug Administration (FDA), among which the third one was only approved this year and found to be effective against the Gram-negative Enterobacteriaceae group for the first time after 1962. Keeping all the above facts of continuous emergence of antibiotic resistance in planktonic bacteria and in their biofilm counterpart, this book chapter has tried to add some more alternative drug resources by means of natural products, which could ultimately lead to the betterment of humankind. Several recent studies have shown that natural products (mainly phytochemicals) exhibit their antibacterial activity through different mechanisms of action like bacterial membrane damage, inhibition of virulence factors, quorum sensing signalling, inhibition of enzymes and toxins. Quorum sensing is a signalling process to regulate the expression of several virulence factors in both Gram-negative and Gram-positive bacteria via an autoinducing loop. When a critical bacterial cell density is reached, a complex of the regulatory proteins and specific signalling molecules enable the autoinduction of the quorum sensor and the expression of the target genes. Quorum sensing inhibitors (QSIs) interfering with this regulatory network have either been derived from natural sources *viz.* phytochemicals and fungi, or they have been chemically synthesized. In this chapter, we will summarize the updates from the available literature describing the various QSIs obtained from natural sources and their role as anti-infective agents. We will also discuss the feasibility of these sources towards the development of future drugs to cure systematic infections in the human body.

**Keywords:** Alternative drug, Antibiotic, Antimicrobial resistance, Anti-infective agent, Infectious disease, Natural product, Pathogen, Quorum sensing, Quorum sensing inhibitor, Virulence factor.

* **Corresponding author Debaprasad Parai:** ICMR-Regional Medical Research Centre, Bhubaneswar, 751023, India;
E-mail: debaprasad.bio@gmail.com

**Parvesh Singh, Vipan Kumar & Rajshekhar Karpoormath (Eds.)**

# ANTIMICROBIAL RESISTANCE AND ITS MECHANISMS

Antimicrobial resistance (AMR) is defined as the inability of the existing drugs to completely eliminate the target microorganisms. After the discovery of the first commercialized antibiotic, penicillin, by Sir Alexander Fleming in 1928, there was no looking back. It was succeeded by some overwhelming discoveries of a wide variety of antibiotics. But eventually, pathogens started developing resistance against existing drugs and later acquired resistance against subsequent newly discovered drugs. The scenario even worsened by the advent of multi-drug resistant (MDR) pathogens which resisted the action of many antibiotics and chemotherapeutic agents. Multi-drug resistance in bacteria occurs by the accumulation of resistance (R) plasmids or transposons, with each gene coding for resistance to a specific agent, and/or by the presence of multidrug efflux pumps which can pump out one or more than one type of drug [1 - 3].

AMR threatens the effective prevention and treatment of an ever-increasing range of infectious microorganisms like bacteria, viruses, parasites and fungi. In nature, antimicrobial resistant organisms are naturally developed with the course of time due to genetic mutations following the natural process of evolution, and then disseminated among humans, animals, food, plants and environment. Among various grounds, some of the common reasons that can lead to the development of AMR are nature's selection pressure, mutation, and horizontal gene transfer (HGT) along with inappropriate use of broad-spectrum antibiotics. It is only in the past few years that gene exchange has been established as a universal property of bacteria that has occurred throughout eons of microbial evolution [4]. Moreover, the importance of HGT in genomic evolution was strengthened by the presence of putative bacterial gene sequences in eukaryotic genomes. Other notable factors contributing to unrestrained occurrences of resistance are identification and distribution of genomic islands carrying genes for pathogenicity along with plasmid-mediated transfer of antibiotic resistance [5]. Most of the bacterial pathogens have evolved into MDR forms with enhanced morbidity and mortality due to high levels of mutation rate [4]. Many MDR strains of *Escherichia coli*, *Staphylococcus aureus*, *Pseudomonas aeruginosa*, *Streptococcus pneumoniae*, *Clostridium difficile*, *Salmonella enterica*, *Mycobacterium tuberculosis*, *Acinetobacter baumannii*, *Klebsiella pneumoniae*, *Neisseria gonorrhoeae* and *Candida auris* have been observed over the past half-century to cause a variety of diseases in humans [6, 7].

AMR is a major threat to public health and leads to economic losses. A global collaborative approach to fight against AMR is required from all concerned sectors that are affected directly or indirectly. The inability to treat common infections is directly rooted with antimicrobial resistance, which, in turn is caused by the emergence and spread of drug-resistant pathogens that have acquired new resistance mechanisms. Unfortunately, the spread of antibiotic resistance is a complex web where the path is interconnected, including the food chain, healthcare facilities and the environment. The rapid spread of multi- and pan-drug resistant bacteria (also known as "superbugs") that cause infections, which are not cured by existing antimicrobials like common antibiotics, is a matter of grave concern. Another outstanding factor that influences and enhances AMR is the occurrence of microbial biofilms [8 - 10]. According to World Health Organization (WHO), with the global rise in AMR, the recalcitrant nature of biofilms is becoming a major concern affecting the healthcare setup, threatening medical procedures, endangering sustainable pharmacological progress and ultimately causing an economical burden. The situation further deteriorates due to the lack of new antimicrobials in the clinical pipeline, lack of access to quality antimicrobials and serious antibiotic shortages affecting entire health-care systems. In 2019, WHO identified 32 antibiotics in clinical development that address the WHO list of priority pathogens, out of which only six were designated to be innovative [11]. The world might be on the inception of a "post antibiotic era," as antibiotics are becoming increasingly ineffective, accompanied by global spread of drug-resistance, which finally ends up producing a more difficult situation in treating infections and causing enormous loss of life. The fundamental approach in treating AMR across the globe primarily lies in the outlook of people towards responsible use of antibiotics [9, 12].

Antimicrobial resistance is reported from all regions of the world. Modern travel of people, animals, and goods accelerates the easy spread of antimicrobial resistance across borders and continents. For example, the rate of resistance towards ciprofloxacin, an antibiotic commonly used to treat urinary tract infections, increased from 8.4% to 92.9% for *E. coli* and from 4.1% to 79.4% for *K. pneumonia*, in countries reporting to the Global Antimicrobial Resistance Surveillance System (GLASS), a program launched to support the global action plan on antimicrobial resistance in collaboration with the WHO AMR Surveillance and Quality Assessment Collaborating Centres Network [13].

## CURRENT UPDATE ON ANTIMICROBIAL RESISTANCE IN CHRONIC BACTERIAL INFECTIONS

The presence of large gaps in the existing surveillance system has restricted the prediction of the exact scenario of antibiotic resistance across the globe. The Centres for Disease Control and Prevention (CDC) and WHO are two global surveillance agencies that work tirelessly to control the introduction and spread of infectious diseases along with providing consultation and assistance to other nations and international agencies to assist in improving their disease prevention and control, environmental health, and health promotion activities. The CDC is a branch of the United States government that answers to the President, Congress and the courts, while the WHO is a United Nations agency and answers to an annual assembly of the world's health ministers. CDC reports that each year at least 2.8 million people get infected with an antibiotic-resistant infection in the U.S. and more than 35,000 people die due to it [14]. In 2013, CDC published its first antibiotic resistance (AR) threats report, which intimated the alarming condition about the danger imposed by antibiotic resistance [7]. The next report issued in 2019 depicted the increasing cases of resistant infections in the community and the number of national deaths caused by it. The three basic goals of the 2019 AR threat report were penned as:

- To serve as a reference for information on antibiotic resistance
- To provide the latest U.S. antibiotic resistance burden estimates for human health
- To highlight emerging areas of concern and areas where additional action is needed

Despite dedicatedly working for the prevention and reduction in the numbers of infections and deaths caused due to AMR, the total number of people affected by antibiotic resistance is still too high. The U.S. government launched a year-long program named as "AMR Challenge" involving more than 350 organizations across the globe to accelerate the fight against AMR [15]. The CDC in its 2018-2019 AMR Challenge focussed on five commitment areas:

- Precise tracking and improvement in AMR data collection
- Prevention and control of infections caused by resistant germs
- Responsible antibiotic use only when needed and prescribed
- Nurturing environment and improving sanitation
- Development of vaccines, therapeutics and diagnostics along with improved access

Surprisingly, CDC's present report shows that there were nearly twice as many annual deaths caused by antibiotic-resistant infections as CDC originally reported in 2013. Therefore, CDC's 2019 report establishes a new national baseline for the number of infections and deaths caused by antibiotic-resistant pathogens. Moreover, the new report categorizes the top antibiotic-resistant threats based on the level of detrimental effect on human health as urgent, serious and concerning. Although there has been significant progress in preventing infections and deaths from resistant organisms typically associated with hospitals, antibiotic-resistant pathogens often found in healthcare setups, including carbapenem-resistant

Enterobacteriaceae (CRE) and methicillin-resistant *S. aureus* (MRSA) which have caused more than 85 percent of the total deaths calculated in the CDC report [14]. CDC is involved in continual inauguration of multiple programs to improve antibiotic use, track resistance and implement infection prevention and control activities in healthcare settings. Among them one such program is "AR Solutions Initiative" in which CDC collaborates with countries where antibiotic resistance can emerge and amplify the spread to investigate and contain resistance outbreaks. In 2019, a new AMR indicator was included in the Sustainable Development Goals (SDG) monitoring framework. The indicator is assigned to monitor the frequency of bloodstream infections caused due to the presence of two specific drug resistant pathogens: MRSA and *E. coli* resistant to third generation cephalosporins. Following which itself in 2019, 25 countries, territories and areas provided data to GLASS on blood-stream infections due to MRSA with a probable median rate of 12.11% and 49 countries provided data on bloodstream infections due to *E. coli* with a probable median rate of 36.0% [11, 13, 16].

Another independent organization working tirelessly along with CDC to combat AMR is WHO. On 29th January, 2018, WHO released its first GLASS report which revealed high levels of resistance to a number of serious bacterial infections. The more distressing finding was that the cases of resistance existed in both high and low-income countries. The report revealed widespread occurrence of antibiotic resistance among 5,00,000 people with suspected bacterial infections across 22 countries. Presently, 52 countries (25 high-income, 20 middle-income and 7 low-income countries) are enrolled in WHO's GLASS program. The most commonly reported resistant bacteria are *E. coli, K. pneumoniae, S. aureus, S. pneumoniae* and *Salmonella* spp. However, the system does not incorporate data on resistance of *M. tuberculosis*, which causes tuberculosis (TB). Among patients with suspected bloodstream infection, the proportion that had bacteria resistant to at least one of the most commonly used antibiotics ranged tremendously between different countries - from 0% to 82%. Yet the data presented in this first GLASS report varied widely in quality and completeness. Furthermore, it has been reported that some countries face major challenges in building their own national surveillance systems. This inability includes lack of personnel, funds and infrastructure. As a result, WHO is supporting more countries to set up their own national antimicrobial resistance surveillance systems that can effectively generate reliable and meaningful data. GLASS is helping to standardize the ways in which countries can collect data and can enliven with a more complete picture about antimicrobial resistance patterns and trends [13].

# QUORUM SENSING AND ITS IMPORTANCE IN BACTERIAL VIRULENCE

Microbial quorum sensing (QS) is a cell-cell communication process that involves small signal molecules which work together to create a hierarchical network of gene regulation in response to microbial population density and alteration in species composition in the adjacent environment. With the concomitant increase in the concentration of the signal molecules as a virtue of the increase in microbial cellular density, a critical concentration is reached, which in turn alters the expression of several target genes. QS signalling systems mainly relied on three principal small molecules namely N-acyl homoserine lactones (AHLs), autoinducing peptides (AIPs) and autoinducer-2 (AI-2) [17 - 19]. This signalling system varies widely in Gram-positive and Gram-negative bacteria with AIP signalling molecules being produced by the Gram-positive bacteria and AHL signalling molecules being produced mainly by Gram-negative bacteria. Both Gram-positive and Gram-negative bacteria produce and use AI-2 signals. These QS signalling systems function in combinations leading to a complex network of regulatory systems that maintain bacterial growth, sustenance and plays an important role in human disease. QS monitors several phenomena such as bioluminescence, regulation of virulence factor gene expression, formation of biofilm, sporulation, swarming and swimming motilities, antibiotic biosynthesis and other biological behaviours [20, 21]. The molecular signalling process has been extensively studied in two important mostly human pathogens, *P. aeruginosa* and *S. aureus*.

Quorum sensing in *P. aeruginosa* comprises three systems that are interconnected in hierarchical order and together govern the expression of hundreds of genes. *Pseudomonas aeruginosa* relies on two AHL dependent QS systems having two pairs of LuxR/I homologs known as LasR/I and RhlR/I, both acting as transcriptional activators in a hierarchical manner. Two AHL ligands, N-(3-oxododecanoyl)-L-homoserine lactone (3O-C12-HSL) and N-butyryl-L-homoserine lactone (C4-HSL) are produced by *lasI* and *rhlI* respectively, which indeed regulate the production of virulence factors *viz.* elastases, proteases, pyocyanin and rhamnolipids via LasR/RhlR binding. Moreover, LasR also regulates LasI expression, which forms a positive feedback loop that rapidly amplifies the amount of LasI to increase the amount of AHLs produced early in the quorum-sensing process [19, 22, 23]. Another type of QS signal molecule, 2-heptyl-3-hydroxy-4-quinolone or *Pseudomonas* quinolone signal (PQS: a product of 2-alkyl-4-quinolone or AHQ family) is produced by *P. aeruginosa* playing a significant role in biofilm development (Fig. **1**). The *pqsABCDE* operon regulates the synthesis and action of PQS genes through a transcriptional regulator PqsR (*mvfR* product) that is further positively controlled by LasR [24]. In addition, PQS binds to the transcriptional regulator MvfR and controls the production of pyocyanin along with RhlR. RsaL binds to *lasI* promoter, prevents LasR mediated activation and thus plays an important role in *las* signalling homeostasis. Other two transcription factors Vfr and VqsR regulate QS-related virulence phenotypes in *P. aeruginosa* [19].

**Fig. (1).** Schematic illustration of QS-mediated virulence factors production and their regulation in *P. aeruginosa*. HHQ: 2-heptyl-4-hydroxyquinolone, AA: Anthranilic acid, PQS: *Pseudomonas* quinolone signal.

In staphylococci, QS is established by the Accessory Gene Regulator (Agr) system, which produces a secreted, post-translationally modified peptide that interacts with a two-component system in an autofeedback loop, ultimately resulting in a considerable shift in gene expression patterns during the early stationary growth phase [25]. The *agr* locus is 3.5 kb in size and consists of two divergent transcriptional units, RNAII and RNAIII, whose transcription is driven by the P2 and P3 promoters, respectively. The RNAII locus contains four genes as *agrB*, *agrD*, *agrC* and *agrA*. AgrD transcript encodes a peptide precursor of the extracellular quorum signal of Agr, known as AIP. The *agrB* gene product is a transmembrane endopeptidase that is responsible for AgrD modification, C-terminal cleavage, and export of the AIP. The *agrC* and *agrA* genes encode a two-component signal transduction system involving a histidine kinase sensor AgrC, which is phosphorylated upon the binding of AIP. Upon being activated by AgrC-dependent phosphorylation, AgrA binds to the P2 promoter region for RNAII and the P3 promoter region for RNAIII. RNAIII is the intracellular effector molecule of the Agr system responsible for the control of Agr targets. It is also a messenger RNA, containing the *hld* gene for delta-hemolysin. In general, Agr upregulates toxins and other acute virulence factors and down-regulates surface proteins (Fig. **2**). In *S. aureus*, the up-regulation of virulence factors by Agr is necessary for disease progression in several animal models of acute infections. Conversely, down-regulation by Agr of phenol-soluble modulins and microbial surface components has been implicated in enhanced biofilm formation and associated virulence. SarA as staphylococci accessory regulator also play significant roles to ensure the establishment of biofilm and biofilm-associated virulence [26 - 29].

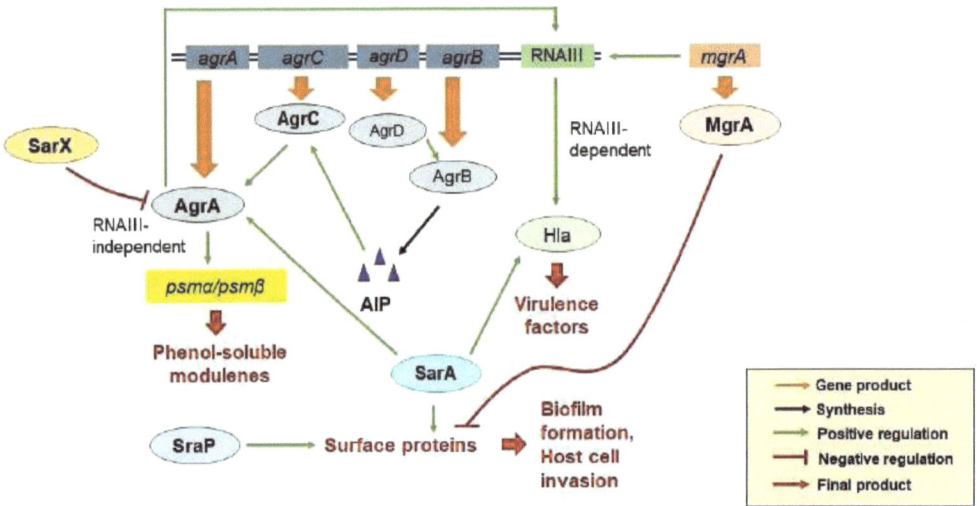

**Fig. (2).** Schematic representation of dynamic and intricate regulatory networks found in *S. aureus* QS system.

## QUORUM SENSING INHIBITORS FROM NATURAL PRODUCTS

In the last couple of decades, there has been a massive imbalance between the emergence of bacterial resistance and the rate of discovery of novel therapeutics. Increasing evidences of AMR has compelled researchers to shift their attention from conventional antibiotics and search for novel next-generation anti-infectives. In the past few years, quorum sensing inhibitors (QSIs) have proved themselves as a promising alternative or potent adjuvants of in-use commercialized antibiotics for the treatment of antibiotic-resistant pathogenic strains of microorganisms. It is supposed that QSIs don't generate selection pressure during attenuation of microbial pathogenicity as compared to the antimicrobial treatments [30]. Interfering with the QS of the target pathogen enables enhanced eradication of the pathogen especially whose virulence system is being regulated by signalling molecules.

There are various ways [31] of inhibiting the QS pathway of the target pathogen which includes:

- inhibition of the synthesis of AI
- antagonism towards AIs receptor
- inhibition of target molecules/genes downstream of receptor binding
- AIs sequestration using various molecules, for example, antibodies against AIs for their sequestration
- AIs degradation using either catalytic antibodies (abzymes) or enzymes (such as lactonases)
- AI secretion/transport inhibition
- administration of antibodies that enfold AIs receptors, finally blocking them.

Therefore, numerous strategies have been chalked out encompassing the hindrance of the QS systems, which can be applied in the control of QS-dependent infections produced by different microbial life-forms. The process of inactivation or degradation of QS signal molecules is known as quorum quenching (QQ), which can be implemented by interfering with the cell-cell communication and monitoring the behaviour of the infectious microorganisms without obstructing their growth. Thus, the phenomenon of antimicrobial resistance can be circumvented but simultaneously the virulence can be curtailed [32, 33]. To summarize the above discussed points, two factors are the centre of discussion, one is the QQ and the other are the QS inhibitory molecules. On one hand, QQ can be efficiently obtained either by the development of antibodies against respective QS signal molecules or by enzymatic inhibition of QS signal molecules or through agents that interfere and block the QS. On the other hand, ideal QS inhibitors are desired to be chemically stable and highly effective with low molecular-mass molecules, exhibiting a high degree of specificity for the QS regulator without cytotoxic effects on the eukaryotic host [31].

Therefore, there is a dire need for the discovery of novel, non-toxic and broad-spectrum anti-QS agents for coping up with the exigency which has arisen due to global antimicrobial resistance. Thus, various natural resources such as phytochemicals, marine microorganisms including marine bacteria and marine fungi along with their derivatives are being explored for their biological activities and therapeutic roles in combating QS of life-threatening pathogens.

## Phytochemicals

Since ancient ages, phytochemicals are reported of possessing therapeutic properties with relatively less cytotoxicity, wide range of chemical diversity and different mechanisms of killing pathogens. Plants have been a persistent source of traditional medicines for their customary usage as a primary medication in both developing and developed countries across the world. Therefore, it was likely that plants might be one of the potential sources for novel QSIs in combating the global scenario of resistance. Phytochemicals are mostly secondary metabolites that possess several benefits along with antimicrobial and antibiofilm properties against pathogenic microbes [34]. Major groups of these plant derived compounds include phenolics, phenolic acids, quinones, saponins, flavonoids, tannins, coumarins, terpenoids, and alkaloids. It is the variation in their chemical and structural composition that makes these compounds vary in their QS inhibitory action. The first reported anti-QS compound was from the benthic marine macroalga *Delisea pulchra* which produced halogenated furanones. The halogenated furanones were found to repress the QS-regulated behaviours by competitively binding with the LuxR type proteins. Thus, biofilm formation was inhibited by enhancing the rate of proteolytic degradation without disturbing the growth of bacteria [35 - 39].

Phytochemicals consumed on a daily basis from various fruits and vegetables such as naringenin, oroidin, salicylic acid, ursolic acid, cinnamaldehyde, methyl eugenol, and garlic are reported to exhibit an anti-biofilm property [40]. For example, embelin and piperine were explored for their anti-biofilm attributes against *Streptococcus mutans*. It was hypothesized that these compounds might interfere with QS pathway to exhibit their antibiofilm effects [41]. Anacardic acids mixture (AAM) isolated from *Amphipterygium adstringens* showed anti-QS potential by restricting QS-controlled virulence factors rhamnolipid, pyocyanin and elastase expressed in *P. aeruginosa*. It reduced 86% of pyocyanin production at 200 μg/mL, 91% of rhamnolipid production at 500 μg/mL and 75% of elastase production at 500 μg/mL in *P. aeruginosa* [42]. Malabaricone C isolated from the bark of *Myristica cinnamomea* impeded QS-regulated violacein production in *Chromobacterium violaceum* CV026 and pyocyanin production along with biofilm formation in *P. aeruginosa* PAO1 [43]. Some phytochemicals inhibit QS-dependent phenotypes in a concentration-dependent manner. Naturally occurring anthocyanin-cyanidin significantly retards biofilm formation, violacein production and EPS production in opportunistic pathogen *K. pneumonia* [44]. Rosmarinic acid obtained from sweet basil shows diverse ways of QS regulation in *P. aeruginosa*. It could bind to the QS-regulator RhlR of *P. aeruginosa* PAO1 and competes with the bacterial ligand C4-HSL. It also escalates biofilm formation and production of the virulence factors like pyocyanin and elastase [45]. Garlic is considered to be a super food with various records of its antibiofilm activity. Even disulphides and trisulphides metabolites, extracted from garlic can inhibit LuxR-based QS genes in *P. aeruginosa* [46]. Various components extracted from grapefruit have shown strong anti-virulence property. A constituent of grapefruit, limonoid has been proven its strong antagonistic activity against both AHL and AI-2 systems, biofilm formation and virulence of enterohemorrhagic *E. coli*. Naturally occurring furocoumarins from grapefruit showed strong repression of AI-1 and AI-2 signal systems in *Vibrio harveyi* and hindrance of biofilm formation in *E. coli*, *Salmonella typhimurium*, and *P. aeruginosa* [46, 47].

The inhibitory action of the flavonoids is wide ranged which might vary from the restricting various cellular functions like gyrase activity, nucleic acid synthesis, type IV topoisomerase, cytoplasmic membrane functions, energy metabolism to obstructing cell-cell communications as observed between rhizobia bacteria and their respective legume hosts during establishment of symbiosis. Flavanones like naringenin, eriodictyol, naringin and taxifolin are reported to significantly reduce the production of pyocyanin, elastase and other virulence factors in *P. aeruginosa* [48 - 50]. Additionally, naringenin and taxifolin were found to decline the expression of several QS-controlled genes such as *lasI*, *lasR*, *rhlI*, *rhlR*, *lasA*, *lasB*, *phzA1*, and *rhlA* in *P. aeruginosa* PAO1 [51]. Another flavonoid called quercetin and tannin showed a significant reduction in several QS-controlled phenotypes such as violacein production, biofilm formation, exopolysaccharide (EPS) production, motility and alginate production in a concentration-dependent manner. Quercetin is found to act as a competitive inhibitor for LasR transcriptional regulator in *P. aeruginosa* and thus significantly curbed biofilm formation along with production of several virulence factors like pyocyanin, protease and elastase [52, 53]. Similarly, *C. albiflorum* (Tul.) Jongkind (*Combretaceae*) derived catechin showed notable reduction in pyocyanin and elastase productions, biofilm formation, along with lowering the expression of the QS-regulated genes *lasB* and *rhlA* and key QS regulatory genes *lasI*, *lasR*, *rhlI* and *rhlR* [54]. Baicalein belongs to the flavone group, which inhibits biofilm formation in *P. aeruginosa* PAO1 at micromolar concentrations and promote proteolysis of the *Agrobacterium tumefaciens* QS-signal receptor TraR in *E. coli* cells at millimolar concentrations. Along with ubiquitous impediment of biofilm formation, flavonoids are also reported to interfere with QS-dependent phenomenon of bioluminescence [31, 55].

There are evidences that diterpene phytol is capable of reducing biofilm formation, twitching and flagellar motility along with significant reduction in pyocyanin production in case of *P. aeruginosa* PAO1 [56]. Alkaloids like reserpine was also found to compete with LasR signal molecule 3O-C12-HSL in *P. aeruginosa* PAO1 and interfere with the production of QS-associated virulence factors [57]. Other significant phytochemicals include carvacrol, which is one of the major antimicrobial components of oregano oil. It inhibits biofilm formation of *C. violaceum* ATCC 12472, *Salmonella enterica* subsp. *Typhimurium* DT104 and *S. aureus* 0074 by reducing the expression of a QS-regulated gene encoding AHL synthase, which is involved in the production of violacein and chitinase [58]. Anthocyanin isolated from *Syzygium cumini* specifically inhibits the violacein production in *C. violaceum* up to an extent of 82%. It also represses biofilm formation and EPS production in *K. pneumoniae* up to a magnitude of 79.94% and 64.29%, respectively [59]. Few more phytochemicals and its mode of actions are given in the Table **1**.

**Table 1. Phytochemicals and its mode of actions.**

| Natural Product | Source | Quorum quenching activity | References |
|---|---|---|---|
| Seaweed extract | *Asparagopsis taxiformis* | Inhibition of violacein | [60] |
| Green alga extract | *Chlamydomonas reinhardtii* | Inhibit QS-regulated luminescence in LasR reporter | [61] |
| Natural pigment | *Auricularia auricular* | Inhibit AHL-inducible violacein production | [62] |
| Metabolite | *Leptolyngbya crossbyana* | Downregulate LasR-regulated elastase production | [63] |
| Emodin | *Rheum palmatum* L. | Accelerate proteolysis of the QS signal receptor TraR, LasR | [64] |
| Plant extract | *Hypericum perforatum* L. | Block the signalling pathway in the Las and Rhl systems | [65] |
| Terpenes and sterols | *Ceiba aesculifolia and C. pentandra* | Attenuate virulence factors and biofilm formation | [66] |
| Curcumin | *Curcuma longa* L. | Inhibit production of pyocyanin, proteases, elastases | [67] |
| Malabaricone C, Giganteone A | *Myristica cinnamomea* | Inhibit pyocyanin production. Reduce bioluminescence expression | [42, 68] |
| Hordenine | *Hordeum vulgare* L. | Reduce gene expression regulated by quorum sensing | [69] |
| Allicin, ajoene | *Allium sativum* L. | Attenuate virulence factors by inhibiting QS genes | [70] |
| Berberine | Plants of *Berberis* genus | Inhibit the expressions of *lasI, lasR, rhlI, rhlR* genes | [71] |
| Parthenolide | *Tanacetum parthenium* L. | Interfere with the binding of AHL to the LasR protein | [72] |
| Salicylic acid | Various plants | Inhibit the expressions of *lasI, lasR, rhlI, rhlR* genes | [73] |

*(Table 1) cont.....*

| Natural Product | Source | Quorum quenching activity | References |
|---|---|---|---|
| Baicalin | *Scutellaria baicalensis* | Inhibit protease, elastase, pyocyanin, rhamnolipid, motilities and exotoxin A | [74] |
| *trans*-anethole | Various species | Interfere with the binding of N-(--oxododecanoyl)-L-homoserine lactone (3O-C$_{12}$-HSL) to the LasR protein | [75] |
| Fruit extract | *Terminalia chebula* | Downregulate expression of LasR/I and RhlR/I systems | [76] |
| Cinnamaldehyde, eugenol | Bark of cinnamon tree | Inhibition of Las and PQS system. Inhibits protease activity and pigment production | [77, 78] |
| Resveratrol | Various species | Inhibit AHL synthesis | [79] |
| Andrographolide | *Andrographis paniculata* | Attenuate Las/Rhl system-controlled virulence factors | [80] |
| Coumarin | Various species | Block QS signalling pathway: Las, PQS and Vsm system | [81] |
| Carvacrol and thymol | *Thymus vulgaris* L. *and* other Lamiaceae species | Reduce the transcriptional levels of *hla*, *sea*, and *seb* genes | [58, 82] |
| Phenolic compounds | Various species | Interfere with CviI/CviR systems of *C. violaceum*. Inhibits AHL production and biofilm formation | [83] |

## Marine Microorganisms

Marine microbial species are considered to be an unexplored reservoir for possessing a wide variety of QSIs, due to their chemical diversity, numerous biological activities and due to the fact that QS is reported to be a frequent phenomenon in marine ecosystems. The promising fact about marine microbes is that they have not been fully exploited yet unlike their terrestrial counterparts. Based on research findings, it has been established that less than 1% of the valuable compounds derived from marine environments have been explored so far, suggesting the very low percentage of metabolites isolated from marine microbial species [30, 84].

### Marine Gram-positive Bacteria

Unique physiological and genetic properties enable halophilic microorganisms to possess a multitude of bioactive secondary metabolites. Two phenethylamide metabolites namely 2,3-methyl-N-(2'-phenylethyl)-butyramide and N-(2--phenylethyl)-isobutyramide, isolated from *Halobacillus salinus* C42 were reported to inhibit QS-regulated violacein biosynthesis of *C. violaceum* CV026 and green fluorescent protein production of *E. coli* JB525 [85]. These two metabolites acted as antagonists of bacterial QS by competing with AHL for receptor binding. Diketopiperazines from microorganisms are seen to possess dual functions, they can either activate or inhibit bacterial QS, pointing to a vital role of these molecules within microbial communities. Archaea are examined for their ability to interact with AHL-producing bacteria in syntrophic communities, such that, cyclo(L-Pro-L-Val) isolated from *Haloterrigena hispanica* SK-3 could promote the expression of QS-regulated genes in bacterial AHL reporters [86]. Contrastingly, four different diketopiperazines- cyclo(L-Pro-L-Phe), cyclo(L-Pr--L-Leu), cyclo(L-Pro-L-isoLeu) and cyclo(L-Pro-D-Phe) isolated from *Marinobacter* sp. SK-3 demonstrated QS-inhibitory activities to *C. violaceum* CV017 and *E. coli* [87]. The first report of the *agr* QS inhibitors from the marine bacteria *Photobacterium* was two novel depsipeptides, solonamide A and B which interfered with *agr* QS activity in a highly virulent, community-acquired strain named *S. aureus* USA300 and *S. aureus* 8325-4 [88]. 2-methyl-N--20-phenylethyl)-butyramide, 3-methyl-N-(20-phenylethyl)-butyramide and benzyl benzoate were three active metabolites from *Oceanobacillus* sp. XC22919 to exhibit the apparent QS inhibitory activities against *C. violaceum* 026 and *P. aeruginosa*. They acted by inhibiting violacein production in *C. violaceum* 026 along with suppression of pyocyanin, elastase and proteolytic enzymes production, and biofilm formation in *P. aeruginosa* [89].

### Marine Gram-Negative Bacteria

Several QSIs have been reported from the marine environment that is being produced by Gram-negative marine bacteria. To mention a few instances, *Gracilaria gracilis* seaweed associated bacteria *Vibrio alginolyticus* G16 shows the capability of disrupting QS signalling pathways along with biofilm formation in *Serratia marcescens*. Virulence factor biosynthesis in *S. marcescens* is inhibited by an active phenol compound named 2,4-bis(1,1-dimethylethyl) which led to the reduction in expression of *bsmA* gene [90]. Simultaneously, this phenol compound could influence hydration of the microbial cell wall along with enhancing the susceptibility of *S. marcescens* towards gentamicin, thereby making it a potential anti-biofilm agent with multiple mode of action and prospective of being used in combinational drug therapy, heightening the efficacy of clinical antibiotics. Another remarkable finding was the isolation of active diketopiperazine, cyclo (Trp–Ser) from the marine bacterium, *Rheinheimera aquimaris* QSI02. It reduced QS-regulated virulence factors production by binding to the LasR receptor with more affinity than natural QS-signalling molecules (AHLs) [91]. MomL, a novel AHL lactonase derived from marine *Muricauda olearia* Th120, also significantly attenuated the production of protease and pyocyanin of *P. aeruginosa* PAO1, without affecting the normal growth of PAO1. AHL accumulation in the cultures were subsequently reduced, pointing towards the fact that AHL degradation resulted in depletion of virulence factor production [92]. QS processes are quite familiar among marine microorganisms and eventually many QSIs are discovered from the marine environments, but QSIs from marine Gram-negative bacteria are still very scanty when compared to marine Gram-positive bacteria. The basic stumbling block might be the problems faced in probing QSIs from marine Gram-negative bacteria using traditional bioassay-guided isolation.

## Marine Fungi and Their Derivatives

As discussed earlier, marine environments are a diverse source of various QSIs due to the presence and contribution of various types of residing marine microbes. Marine fungi are one of them, which are known to be dynamic producers of many QSIs due to their ability of synthesizing and secreting diverse secondary metabolites, such as polyketide-derived alkaloids, terpenes, peptides and mixed biosynthesis metabolites [93]. Equisetin is one such QSI, derived from a marine fungus *Fusarium* sp. Z10, which attenuates biofilm formation and many QS-regulated activities such as swarming motility, LasR/I, RhlR/I and the PQS system of *P. aeruginosa*. Further studies showed that equisetin could inhibit the production of various virulence factors such as elastin, pyocyanin. The compound acts restricting the transcriptional activation of LasB in *E. coli* MG4/pKDT17 along with transcriptional activation of PqsA in *E. coli* pEAL08-2, with decline in rhamnolipid biosynthesis, swarming motility and transcriptional activation of RhlA in *E. coli* pDSY [94]. Kojic acid is a pyrone derivative from marine-derived fungus *Altenaria* sp. of host alga *Ulva pertusa*, attenuated QS-dependent luminescence of *E. coli* pSB401 orchestrated by N-hexanoyl-L-homoserine lactone (C6-HSL) [95]. Asteltoxin is a reported QS inhibitor from marine fungus *Penicillium* sp. QF046, which exhibits more robust suppression of violacein production and has decreased expression of multiple QS-related genes namely *lasA*, *lasB*, *cynS*, *hcnB*, *vioB*, and *vioI* [30]. Six QSIs has been isolation from secondary metabolites of *Penicillium* sp. SCS-KFD08 when tested against *C. violaceum* CV026. Among these six isolated QSIs, two compounds inhibited violacein biosynthesis in *C. violaceum* CV026 up to an extent of 46% and 49% respectively at sub-minimal inhibitory concentration [96]. Four strains of endophytic fungi belonging to *Sarocladium* (LAEE06), *Fusarium* (LAEE13), *Epicoccum* (LAEE14), and *Khuskia* (LAEE21) exhibit considerable QS inhibiting activity at concentrations ranging between 50 to 500 µg/mL. Two major components variecolorin N and phenylahistin isolated from *Epicoccum* were known to act as QS agonists or antagonists [91].

## MODES OF ACTION OF QSIS

Bacterial QS signals are involved in the regulation of various physiological processes such as virulence factors production, biofilm formation, plasmid conjugation, motility, antibiotic resistance, and thus critically regulate pathogenicity of human pathogens [97]. QSIs are employed to break this cellular hierarchical communication between adjacent microbial cells within host system such that the pathogens become more vulnerable to be cleared by the host immune system. Some of the anti-QS strategies are discussed below that validate the fact that QS are potent therapeutic target for tackling dreadful bacterial diseases:

### Inactivation of QS Receptor

The fundamental objective in a QS signalling system is the binding of the ligand with their respective receptor. Therefore, it is quite obvious that inactivating these receptors in QS signalling is an effective strategy for breaking the QS network and thereby reducing bacterial virulence and infection. Flavonoids are reported to bind with the QS receptors and significantly reduce the expression of virulence genes in *P. aeruginosa* [57, 98]. Similarly, N-decanoyl-L-homoserine benzyl ester is a structural analogue of AHL signals, has been established to reduce the production of virulence factors like elastase and rhamnolipid in *P. aeruginosa*, by blocking their homologous receptors [99]. Unlike receptor analogue, although the mode of action of receptor antagonists varies, they also aim to hinder the QS regulatory system by enhancing the antibacterial activity of various antibiotics and minimizing the therapeutic dose of antibiotics for *P. aeruginosa* infection [100]. AHLs analogs bind with the LuxR receptors in *Vibrio fischeri*, TraR in *A. tumefaciens*, and LasR in case of *P. aeruginosa*. But their unstable nature and tendency to degrade within alkaline conditions restricts the practical application of receptor inhibitors for treating bacterial diseases [101].

### Inhibition of QS Signals Synthesis

Inhibition of AHL synthesis is a direct strategy to reduce AHL-mediated virulence factors and prevent pathological damage. Such is observed in case of sinefungin, butyryl-SAM and S-adenosylhomocysteine, which attenuate the secretion of QS-mediated virulence factors and prevent the bacterial infection by inhibiting the AHL synthesis in *P. aeruginosa* [102, 103]. Similarly, immucillin A and its derivatives was reported to reduce the AHL synthesis by inhibiting the 5-MTAN/S-adenosylhomocysteine nucleosidase [104]. Even triclosan has been documented of reducing AHL synthesis by inhibiting the production of enoyl-ACP reductase precursors [105]. However, the anti-QS agents that inhibit AHL synthesis, also obstruct the metabolism of amino acid and fatty acid having basic role in bacterial nutrition. In the long run, blocking of triclosan on the metabolism of amino acid and fatty acid in the bacteria could develope antibiotic-resistance in *P. aeruginosa* [106]. Thus, drugs specifically inhibiting the AHL synthesis without interfering with the nutritional metabolism of bacteria should be developed for sustainable clinical application.

## Degradation of QS signals

This particular approach is much more convenient because it involves degradation of the QS signals by specific enzymes and also suggested not to cause any selective pressure on the bacteria. The enzymes that are applied for QS signal degradation are lactonase, acylase, oxidoreductases and 3-Hydroxy-2-metyl-4(1H)-quinolone 2, 4- dioxygenase. For example, AHL lactonase is a AHL degrading enzyme of the metallo-$\beta$-lactamase superfamily which is able to prevent bacterial infection by degrading AHLs with different side chain length. AHL lactonases mainly act by increasing the bacterial sensitivity towards antibiotics without affecting the growth of the bacteria as observed in *P. aeruginosa* and *A. baumannii* [107, 108]. This phenomenon is further confirmed by the synergistic action of AHL lactonase and antibiotics in the mice model infected with *P. aeruginosa*, where drugs containing AHL lactonase can effectively inhibit the spread of skin pathogens while minimizing the effective dose of antibiotics. The AHL lactonase is also reported to block biofilm formation in *P. aeruginosa*. Specific AHL lactonase like AiiK produced by engineered *E. coli* is capable of attenuating extracellular proteolytic activity and pyocyanin production in *P. aeruginosa* PAO1 [109, 110]. Another enzyme called the acylase, initially found in *Variovorax paradoxus* and *Ralstonia,* suppresses the QS signalling by hydrolyzing the amide bond of AHLs. The acylase has a wide range of applications starting from attenuating the growth pathogens to commercial application in human health care in the form of an acylase coated device to acting as an antifouling agent [111, 112]. Oxidoreductases are a class of enzymes that can alter the AHL's specificity of homologous intracellular receptors by modifying acyl side chains, leading to a blockage of the expression of QS related virulence genes. For example, BpiB09 oxidoreductase curbs the activation of 3O-C12-HSL in the *P. aeruginosa* PAO1, eventually supressing bacterial motility, biofilms formation, and pyocyanin secretion [113]. Like acylase, oxidoreductases can be immobilized on the glass surface to attenuate biofilm formation *Klebsiella oxytoca* and decrease the growth rate of *K. pneumoniae* [114]. The next discussed enzyme is dioxygenase which can block the quinolone signals in the QS system of *P. aeruginosa* [115]. Dioxygenase has the capability to degrade 2-heptyl-3-hydroxy-4(1H)-quinolone mediated signals and hinder the accumulation of the signalling molecules which in turn reduce the secretion of QS-regulated virulence factors such as pyocyanin, rhamnolipid, and lectin A toxin [116]. These degrading enzymes are potential to be used as alternatives to antibiotics that can be used not only to control bacterial infection but also to minimize the risk of AMR. The only limitation is *in vivo* stability of these enzymes, which impose a great difficulty for their use in biomedical applications.

## Combined Application of Anti-QS Agents and Antibiotics

Combinational studies have always been used in combating critical cases of infections where a single therapeutic was unable to combat with life-threatening pathogens. Subsequently, QSI agents were combined with antibiotics for an effective clinical strategy for the treatment of bacterial diseases [117 - 119]. Many studies have confirmed the synergistic effect of antibiotics and QSI agents. Ajoene, furanone C-30, and horseradish extract have been reported to reduce the expression of virulence factors in *P. aeruginosa*, making it more susceptible to subsequent antibiotic treatment [120 - 122]. Synergistic effects were further confirmed from the combined application of curcumin with gentamicin and azithromycin on *P. aeruginosa*, whereby the expressions of virulence genes were significantly down-regulated by the use of curcumin, lowering the therapeutic dosages of tested antibiotics [123]. Similarly, gallocatechin-3-gallate and caffeic acid, sensitized *Mycoplasma pneumoniae* towards the action of tetracycline, ciprofloxacin and gentamicin [124]. Recent studies showed that both farnesol and hamamelitannin can increase the sensitivity of *S. aureus* to $\beta$-lactam antibiotics by decreasing their virulence factors [125]. These findings imply that combined use of antibiotics with QSI agents has great therapeutic potential against several bacterial diseases.

## FUTURE PERSPECTIVE

The QS system orchestrates the genetically controlled bacterial communication during thedisease establishment within the host. So, one of the effective strategies can be taken by interfering the signalling pathway and eventually restricting their pathogenicity. Common but unexplored natural sources like phytochemicals and marine microorganisms are particularly of immense interest in sustainable management of life-threatening bacterial infections along with lowering the risk of bacterial resistance. Searching for a new alternative against antibiotic-resistant infections, naturally derived QSIs could be a great boon to us, although they have some limitations in terms of selectivity, virulence reduction and lack of resistance against QQ. Signal molecules generally associated with pathogenicity also regulate some of the rarely discussed vital physiological processes of microbes such as metabolism, DNA repair, resistance to stressors, cell division and morphogenesis [126]. Inhibiting these signal molecules could interfere with normal microbial homeostatic and also restrain microbial-host interaction. In some cases, the use of anti-QS therapies could promote the development of isolates with increased pathogenicity, such as deletion of luxS (ΔluxS) was reported to increase the aggregation or/and biofilm formation in *Helicobacter pylori* [127]. QS inhibitors were reported to target QS genes, eventually disrupting the pathogenicity of the microorganisms without exhibiting any bactericidal activity. But contrary to the existing notion, resistance to QS inhibitors were initially reported by *in silico* modelling studies which was later confirmed by *in vitro* studies in *P. aeruginosa* by mutating genes encoding efflux pumps, proteins responsible for the removal of harmful substances from cells [121].

To date, most of research studies with QSIs are done either *in vitro* or in various infected animal models. Unlike *in vitro* QQ activity, *in vivo* QQ activities have a contrasting facet with a different impact on host health. AI-2 was reported to have significant effect on the intestinal microflora of antibiotic-treated mice, whereby the modified *E. coli* strain producing AI-2 promoted the expansion of the *Firmicutes* phylum which in turn increased the *Firmicutes/Bacteroides* ratio in mice guts. It was also observed that the use of antibiotics might most likely contribute to the destruction of microorganisms belonging to *Firmicutes* and created an environment with a low AI-2 concentration [128]. The notable influence of these autoinducers was further demonstrated in anti-QS treated stool samples by calculating the number of *Firmicutes* [129]. Limiting the optimal concentration of QS signals by QQ activity, emergences of pro-inflammatory diseases were reported in the host system. For example, a decrease in the number of butyrate-producing *Clostridium* clade XIVa (which constituted almost 60% of the mucosa-associated gut microbiota) lead to the development of pro-inflammatory diseases such as cystic fibrosis, sclerosis, irritable bowel disease, along with an increase in the number of *Enterococcus* and *C. difficile* in the intestines. The QQ activity not only interferes with the metabolic activity of the host microbiota but also disturbs the signalling factors of the host. AHLs are reported to possess diverse functions in eukaryotic host systems, for instance, they are chemoattractant for neutrophils, induce pro-inflammatory and pro-apoptotic responses, stimulate protective and innate immune responses [130]. Currently, a handful of QSIs are in their preclinical phase and require more clinical trials. Another drawback is their unstable natures and lack of detailed pharmacological studies. However, combinational therapy using QSI agents along with conventional antibiotics holds robust potential in terms of application as it will be able to improve the efficacy of therapeutic drugs and decrease the cost of human healthcare.

## CONSENT FOR PUBLICATION

Not applicable.

## CONFLICT OF INTEREST

The authors declare no conflict of interest, financial or otherwise.

## ACKNOWLEDGEMENTS

Declared none.

## REFERENCES

[1]     Nikaido H. Multidrug resistance in bacteria. Annu Rev Biochem 2009; 78: 119-46.
        [http://dx.doi.org/10.1146/annurev.biochem.78.082907.145923] [PMID: 19231985]

[2]     WHO. Global action plan on antimicrobial resistance. Geneva: World Health Organization 2015; pp. 1-28.

[3]     Tenover FC. Mechanisms of antimicrobial resistance in bacteria. Am J Infect Control 2006; 34(5) (Suppl. 1): S3-S10.
        [http://dx.doi.org/10.1016/j.ajic.2006.05.219] [PMID: 16813980]

[4]     Davies J, Davies D. Origins and evolution of antibiotic resistance. Microbiol Mol Biol Rev 2010; 74(3): 417-33.
        [http://dx.doi.org/10.1128/MMBR.00016-10] [PMID: 20805405]

[5]     Hacker J, Kaper JB. Pathogenicity islands and the evolution of microbes. Annu Rev Microbiol 2000; 54: 641-79.
        [http://dx.doi.org/10.1146/annurev.micro.54.1.641] [PMID: 11018140]

[6]     WHO. Antimicrobial resistance: global report on surveillance. Geneva: World Health Organization 2014.

[7]     CDC. Antibiotic resistance threats in the United States, 2013. Atlanta, GA: U.S. Department of Health and Human Services, CDC 2013.

[8]     Ventola CL. The antibiotic resistance crisis: part 1: causes and threats. P&T 2015; 40(4): 277-83.
        [PMID: 25859123]

[9]     Alanis AJ. Resistance to antibiotics: are we in the post-antibiotic era? Arch Med Res 2005; 36(6): 697-705.
        [http://dx.doi.org/10.1016/j.arcmed.2005.06.009] [PMID: 16216651]

[10]    Michael CA, Dominey-Howes D, Labbate M. The antimicrobial resistance crisis: causes, consequences, and management. Front Public Health 2014; 2: 145.
        [http://dx.doi.org/10.3389/fpubh.2014.00145] [PMID: 25279369]

[11]    Antimicrobial resistance. World Health Organization. Available from: https://www.who.int/news-room/fact-sheets/detail/antimicrobial-resistance

[12]    WHO. WHO report on surveillance of antibiotic consumption: 2016-2018 early implementation 2018.

[13]    WHO. Global antimicrobial resistance surveillance system (GLASS) report: early implementation 2017-2018 2018.

[14]    CDC. Antibiotic resistance threats in the United States. Atlanta, GA: U.S. Department of Health and Human Services, CDC 2019.

[15]    The AMR Challenge. Centers for Disease Control and Prevention. Available from: https://www.cdc.gov/drugresistance/intl-activities/amr-challenge.html

[16]    Antibiotic Resistance: A Global Threat. Available from: https://www.cdc.gov/drugresistance/solutions-initiative/stories/ar-global-threat.html

[17]    Ng W-L, Bassler BL. Bacterial quorum-sensing network architectures. Annu Rev Genet 2009; 43: 197-222.
[http://dx.doi.org/10.1146/annurev-genet-102108-134304] [PMID: 19686078]

[18]    Jiang Q, Chen J, Yang C, Yin Y, Yao K. Quorum sensing: A prospective therapeutic target for bacterial diseases. BioMed Res Int 2019.
[http://dx.doi.org/10.1155/2019/2015978]

[19]    Balasubramanian D, Schneper L, Kumari H, Mathee K. A dynamic and intricate regulatory network determines *Pseudomonas aeruginosa* virulence. Nucleic Acids Res 2013; 41(1): 1-20.
[http://dx.doi.org/10.1093/nar/gks1039] [PMID: 23143271]

[20]    Williams P, Winzer K, Chan WC, Cámara M. Look who's talking: communication and quorum sensing in the bacterial world. Philos Trans R Soc Lond B Biol Sci 2007; 362(1483): 1119-34.
[http://dx.doi.org/10.1098/rstb.2007.2039] [PMID: 17360280]

[21]    Rutherford ST, Bassler BL. Bacterial quorum sensing: its role in virulence and possibilities for its control. Cold Spring Harb Perspect Med 2012; 2(11): a012427.
[http://dx.doi.org/10.1101/cshperspect.a012427] [PMID: 23125205]

[22]    Wagner VE, Li LL, Isabella VM, Iglewski BH. Analysis of the hierarchy of quorum-sensing regulation in *Pseudomonas aeruginosa*. Anal Bioanal Chem 2007; 387(2): 469-79.
[http://dx.doi.org/10.1007/s00216-006-0964-6] [PMID: 17139483]

[23]    Schuster M, Greenberg EP. A network of networks: quorum-sensing gene regulation in *Pseudomonas aeruginosa*. Int J Med Microbiol 2006; 296(2-3): 73-81.
[http://dx.doi.org/10.1016/j.ijmm.2006.01.036] [PMID: 16476569]

[24]    Dubern J-F, Diggle SP. Quorum sensing by 2-alkyl-4-quinolones in *Pseudomonas aeruginosa* and other bacterial species. Mol Biosyst 2008; 4(9): 882-8.
[http://dx.doi.org/10.1039/b803796p] [PMID: 18704225]

[25]    Le KY, Otto M. Quorum-sensing regulation in staphylococci-an overview. Front Microbiol 2015; 6: 1174.
[http://dx.doi.org/10.3389/fmicb.2015.01174] [PMID: 26579084]

[26]    Yarwood JM, Bartels DJ, Volper EM, Greenberg EP. Quorum sensing in *Staphylococcus aureus* biofilms. J Bacteriol 2004; 186(6): 1838-50.
[http://dx.doi.org/10.1128/JB.186.6.1838-1850.2004] [PMID: 14996815]

[27]    Foster TJ, Geoghegan JA, Ganesh VK, Höök M. Adhesion, invasion and evasion: the many functions of the surface proteins of *Staphylococcus aureus*. Nat Rev Microbiol 2014; 12(1): 49-62.
[http://dx.doi.org/10.1038/nrmicro3161] [PMID: 24336184]

[28]    Beenken KE, Dunman PM, McAleese F, *et al.* Global gene expression in *Staphylococcus aureus* biofilms. J Bacteriol 2004; 186(14): 4665-84.
[http://dx.doi.org/10.1128/JB.186.14.4665-4684.2004] [PMID: 15231800]

[29]    López D, Vlamakis H, Kolter R. Biofilms. Cold Spring Harb Perspect Biol 2010; 2(7): a000398.
[http://dx.doi.org/10.1101/cshperspect.a000398] [PMID: 20519345]

[30]    Chen J, Wang B, Lu Y, *et al.* Quorum sensing inhibitors from marine microorganisms and their synthetic derivatives. Mar Drugs 2019; 17(2): 80.
[http://dx.doi.org/10.3390/md17020080] [PMID: 30696031]

[31]    Asfour HZ. Anti-quorum sensing natural compounds. J Microsc Ultrastruct 2018; 6(1): 1-10.
[http://dx.doi.org/10.4103/JMAU.JMAU_10_18] [PMID: 30023261]

[32]    Rasmussen TB, Bjarnsholt T, Skindersoe ME, *et al.* Screening for quorum-sensing inhibitors (QSI) by use of a novel genetic system, the QSI selector. J Bacteriol 2005; 187(5): 1799-814.
[http://dx.doi.org/10.1128/JB.187.5.1799-1814.2005] [PMID: 15716452]

[33]    Rasmussen TB, Givskov M. Quorum-sensing inhibitors as anti-pathogenic drugs. Int J Med Microbiol

2006; 296(2-3): 149-61.
[http://dx.doi.org/10.1016/j.ijmm.2006.02.005] [PMID: 16503194]

[34]   Choo JH, Rukayadi Y, Hwang JK. Inhibition of bacterial quorum sensing by vanilla extract. Lett Appl Microbiol 2006; 42(6): 637-41.
[http://dx.doi.org/10.1111/j.1472-765X.2006.01928.x] [PMID: 16706905]

[35]   Cowan MM. Plant products as antimicrobial agents. Clin Microbiol Rev 1999; 12(4): 564-82.
[http://dx.doi.org/10.1128/CMR.12.4.564] [PMID: 10515903]

[36]   Muhammad Sajid Arshad, Syeda Ayesha Batool. Natural antimicrobials, their sources and food safety, food additives. Desiree Nedra Karunaratne and Geethi Pamunuwa, IntechOpen 2017.

[37]   Saleem M, Nazir M, Ali MS, *et al.* Antimicrobial natural products: an update on future antibiotic drug candidates. Nat Prod Rep 2010; 27(2): 238-54.
[http://dx.doi.org/10.1039/B916096E] [PMID: 20111803]

[38]   Dewick PM 3rd Edition.. Medicinal natural products. A biosynthetic approach 2002.

[39]   Packiavathy IASV, Agilandeswari P, Musthafa KS, Pandian SK, Ravi AV. Antibiofilm and quorum sensing inhibitory potential of *Cuminum cyminum* and its secondary metabolite methyl eugenol against Gram negative bacterial pathogens. Food Res Int 2012; 45: 85-92.
[http://dx.doi.org/10.1016/j.foodres.2011.10.022]

[40]   Dwivedi D, Singh V. Effects of the natural compounds embelin and piperine on the biofilm-producing property of *Streptococcus mutans*. J Tradit Complement Med 2015; 6(1): 57-61.
[http://dx.doi.org/10.1016/j.jtcme.2014.11.025] [PMID: 26870681]

[41]   Castillo-Juárez I, García-Contreras R, Velázquez-Guadarrama N, Soto-Hernández M, Martínez-Vázquez M. Amphypterygium adstringens anacardic acid mixture inhibits quorum sensing-controlled virulence factors of *Chromobacterium violaceum* and *Pseudomonas aeruginosa*. Arch Med Res 2013; 44(7): 488-94.
[http://dx.doi.org/10.1016/j.arcmed.2013.10.004] [PMID: 24126126]

[42]   Chong YM, Yin WF, Ho CY, *et al.* Malabaricone C from *Myristica cinnamomea* exhibits anti-quorum sensing activity. J Nat Prod 2011; 74(10): 2261-4.
[http://dx.doi.org/10.1021/np100872k] [PMID: 21910441]

[43]   Gopu V, Shetty PH. Cyanidin inhibits quorum signalling pathway of a food borne opportunistic pathogen. J Food Sci Technol 2016; 53(2): 968-76.
[http://dx.doi.org/10.1007/s13197-015-2031-9] [PMID: 27162376]

[44]   Corral-Lugo A, Daddaoua A, Ortega A, Espinosa-Urgel M, Krell T. Rosmarinic acid is a homoserine lactone mimic produced by plants that activates a bacterial quorum-sensing regulator. Sci Signal 2016; 9(409): ra1.
[http://dx.doi.org/10.1126/scisignal.aaa8271] [PMID: 26732761]

[45]   Li WR, Ma YK, Xie XB, *et al.* Diallyl disulfide from garlic oil inhibits *Pseudomonas aeruginosa* quorum sensing systems and corresponding virulence factors. Front Microbiol 2019; 9: 3222.
[http://dx.doi.org/10.3389/fmicb.2018.03222] [PMID: 30666240]

[46]   Girennavar B, Cepeda ML, Soni KA, *et al.* Grapefruit juice and its furocoumarins inhibits autoinducer signaling and biofilm formation in bacteria. Int J Food Microbiol 2008; 125(2): 204-8.
[http://dx.doi.org/10.1016/j.ijfoodmicro.2008.03.028] [PMID: 18504060]

[47]   Vikram A, Jesudhasan PR, Jayaprakasha GK, Pillai BS, Patil BS. Grapefruit bioactive limonoids modulate *E. coli* O157:H7 TTSS and biofilm. Int J Food Microbiol 2010; 140(2-3): 109-16.
[http://dx.doi.org/10.1016/j.ijfoodmicro.2010.04.012] [PMID: 20471125]

[48]   Buer CS, Imin N, Djordjevic MA. Flavonoids: new roles for old molecules. J Integr Plant Biol 2010; 52(1): 98-111.
[http://dx.doi.org/10.1111/j.1744-7909.2010.00905.x] [PMID: 20074144]

[49]    Cushnie TP, Lamb AJ. Antimicrobial activity of flavonoids. Int J Antimicrob Agents 2005; 26(5): 343-56.
[http://dx.doi.org/10.1016/j.ijantimicag.2005.09.002] [PMID: 16323269]

[50]    Dey P, Parai D, Banerjee M, Hossain ST, Mukherjee SK. Naringin sensitizes the antibiofilm effect of ciprofloxacin and tetracycline against *Pseudomonas aeruginosa* biofilm. Int J Med Microbiol 2020; 310(3): 151410.
[http://dx.doi.org/10.1016/j.ijmm.2020.151410] [PMID: 32057619]

[51]    Vandeputte OM, Kiendrebeogo M, Rasamiravaka T, *et al.* The flavanone naringenin reduces the production of quorum sensing-controlled virulence factors in Pseudomonas aeruginosa PAO1. Microbiology 2011; 157(Pt 7): 2120-32.
[http://dx.doi.org/10.1099/mic.0.049338-0] [PMID: 21546585]

[52]    Ouyang J, Sun F, Feng W, *et al.* Quercetin is an effective inhibitor of quorum sensing, biofilm formation and virulence factors in *Pseudomonas aeruginosa.* J Appl Microbiol 2016; 120(4): 966-74.
[http://dx.doi.org/10.1111/jam.13073] [PMID: 26808465]

[53]    Lee J-H, Park J-H, Cho HS, Joo SW, Cho MH, Lee J. Anti-biofilm activities of quercetin and tannic acid against *Staphylococcus aureus.* Biofouling 2013; 29(5): 491-9.
[http://dx.doi.org/10.1080/08927014.2013.788692] [PMID: 23668380]

[54]    Vandeputte OM, Kiendrebeogo M, Rajaonson S, *et al.* Identification of catechin as one of the flavonoids from *Combretum albiflorum* bark extract that reduces the production of quorum-sensin--controlled virulence factors in *Pseudomonas aeruginosa* PAO1. Appl Environ Microbiol 2010; 76(1): 243-53.
[http://dx.doi.org/10.1128/AEM.01059-09] [PMID: 19854927]

[55]    Vikram A, Jayaprakasha GK, Jesudhasan PR, Pillai SD, Patil BS. Suppression of bacterial cell-cell signalling, biofilm formation and type III secretion system by citrus flavonoids. J Appl Microbiol 2010; 109(2): 515-27.
[http://dx.doi.org/10.1111/j.1365-2672.2010.04677.x] [PMID: 20163489]

[56]    Pejin B, Ciric A, Glamoclija J, Nikolic M, Sokovic M. *In vitro* anti-quorum sensing activity of phytol. Nat Prod Res 2015; 29(4): 374-7.
[http://dx.doi.org/10.1080/14786419.2014.945088] [PMID: 25103916]

[57]    Parai D, Banerjee M, Dey P, Chakraborty A, Islam E, Mukherjee SK. Effect of reserpine on *Pseudomonas aeruginosa* quorum sensing mediated virulence factors and biofilm formation. Biofouling 2018; 34(3): 320-34.
[http://dx.doi.org/10.1080/08927014.2018.1437910] [PMID: 29482361]

[58]    Burt SA, Ojo-Fakunle VT, Woertman J, Veldhuizen EJ. The natural antimicrobial carvacrol inhibits quorum sensing in *Chromobacterium violaceum* and reduces bacterial biofilm formation at sub-lethal concentrations. PLoS One 2014; 9(4): e93414.
[http://dx.doi.org/10.1371/journal.pone.0093414] [PMID: 24691035]

[59]    Gopu V, Kothandapani S, Shetty PH. Quorum quenching activity of *Syzygium cumini* (L.) Skeels and its anthocyanin malvidin against *Klebsiella pneumoniae.* Microb Pathog 2015; 79: 61-9.
[http://dx.doi.org/10.1016/j.micpath.2015.01.010] [PMID: 25637095]

[60]    Jha B, Kavita K, Westphal J, Hartmann A, Schmitt-Kopplin P. Quorum sensing inhibition by *Asparagopsis taxiformis*, a marine macro alga: separation of the compound that interrupts bacterial communication. Mar Drugs 2013; 11(1): 253-65.
[http://dx.doi.org/10.3390/md11010253] [PMID: 23344114]

[61]    Teplitski M, Chen H, Rajamani S, *et al. Chlamydomonas reinhardtii* secretes compounds that mimic bacterial signals and interfere with quorum sensing regulation in bacteria. Plant Physiol 2004; 134(1): 137-46.
[http://dx.doi.org/10.1104/pp.103.029918] [PMID: 14671013]

[62]   Zhu H, He CC, Chu QH. Inhibition of quorum sensing in *Chromobacterium violaceum* by pigments
       extracted from *Auricularia auricular*. Lett Appl Microbiol 2011; 52(3): 269-74.
       [http://dx.doi.org/10.1111/j.1472-765X.2010.02993.x] [PMID: 21204879]

[63]   Saurav K, Costantino V, Venturi V, Steindler L. Quorum sensing inhibitors from the sea discovered
       using bacterial N-acyl-homoserine lactone-based biosensors. Mar Drugs 2017; 15(3): 53.
       [http://dx.doi.org/10.3390/md15030053] [PMID: 28241461]

[64]   Ding X, Yin B, Qian L, *et al.* Screening for novel quorum-sensing inhibitors to interfere with the
       formation of *Pseudomonas aeruginosa* biofilm. J Med Microbiol 2011; 60(Pt 12): 1827-34.
       [http://dx.doi.org/10.1099/jmm.0.024166-0] [PMID: 21852522]

[65]   Doğan Ş, Gökalsın B, Şenkardeş İ, Doğan A, Sesal NC. Anti-quorum sensing and anti-biofilm
       activities of *Hypericum perforatum* extracts against *Pseudomonas aeruginosa*. J Ethnopharmacol
       2019; 235: 293-300.
       [http://dx.doi.org/10.1016/j.jep.2019.02.020] [PMID: 30763694]

[66]   Muñoz-Cázares N, Aguilar-Rodríguez S, García-Contreras R, *et al.* Phytochemical screening and
       antivirulence properties of *Ceiba pentandra* and *Ceiba aesculifolia* (Malvaceae) bark extracts and
       fractions. Bot Sci 2018; 96: 415-25.
       [http://dx.doi.org/10.17129/botsci.1902]

[67]   Rudrappa T, Bais HP. Curcumin, a known phenolic from *Curcuma longa*, attenuates the virulence of
       *Pseudomonas aeruginosa* PAO1 in whole plant and animal pathogenicity models. J Agric Food Chem
       2008; 56(6): 1955-62.
       [http://dx.doi.org/10.1021/jf072591j] [PMID: 18284200]

[68]   Sivasothy Y, Krishnan T, Chan KG, *et al.* Quorum sensing inhibitory activity of Giganteone A from
       *Myristica cinnamomea* King against *Escherichia coli* biosensors. Molecules 2016; 21(3): 391.
       [http://dx.doi.org/10.3390/molecules21030391] [PMID: 27102164]

[69]   Zhou JW, Luo HZ, Jiang H, Jian TK, Chen ZQ, Jia AQ. Hordenine: a novel quorum sensing inhibitor
       and antibiofilm agent against *Pseudomonas aeruginosa*. J Agric Food Chem 2018; 66(7): 1620-8.
       [http://dx.doi.org/10.1021/acs.jafc.7b05035] [PMID: 29353476]

[70]   Bjarnsholt T, Jensen PØ, Rasmussen TB, *et al.* Garlic blocks quorum sensing and promotes rapid
       clearing of pulmonary *Pseudomonas aeruginosa* infections. Microbiology 2005; 151(Pt 12): 3873-80.
       [http://dx.doi.org/10.1099/mic.0.27955-0] [PMID: 16339933]

[71]   Li Y, Huang J, Li L, Liu L. Synergistic activity of berberine with azithromycin against *Pseudomonas
       aeruginosa* isolated from patients with cystic fibrosis of lung *in vitro* and *in vivo*. Cell Physiol
       Biochem 2017; 42(4): 1657-69.
       [http://dx.doi.org/10.1159/000479411] [PMID: 28738346]

[72]   Kalia M, Yadav VK, Singh PK, Sharma D, Narvi SS, Agarwal V. Exploring the impact of
       parthenolide as anti-quorum sensing and anti-biofilm agent against *Pseudomonas aeruginosa*. Life Sci
       2018; 199: 96-103.
       [http://dx.doi.org/10.1016/j.lfs.2018.03.013] [PMID: 29524516]

[73]   Ahmed SAKS, Rudden M, Smyth TJ, Dooley JSG, Marchant R, Banat IM. Natural quorum sensing
       inhibitors effectively downregulate gene expression of *Pseudomonas aeruginosa* virulence factors.
       Appl Microbiol Biotechnol 2019; 103(8): 3521-35.
       [http://dx.doi.org/10.1007/s00253-019-09618-0] [PMID: 30852658]

[74]   Luo J, Dong B, Wang K, *et al.* Baicalin inhibits biofilm formation, attenuates the quorum sensing-
       controlled virulence and enhances *Pseudomonas aeruginosa* clearance in a mouse peritoneal implant
       infection model. PLoS One 2017; 12(4): e0176883.
       [http://dx.doi.org/10.1371/journal.pone.0176883] [PMID: 28453568]

[75]   Hançer Aydemir D, Çifci G, Aviyente V, Boşgelmez-Tinaz G. Quorum-sensing inhibitor potential of
       trans-anethole aganist Pseudomonas aeruginosa. J Appl Microbiol 2018; 125(3): 731-9.

[http://dx.doi.org/10.1111/jam.13892] [PMID: 29694695]

[76]    Sarabhai S, Sharma P, Capalash N. Ellagic acid derivatives from *Terminalia chebula* Retz. downregulate the expression of quorum sensing genes to attenuate *Pseudomonas aeruginosa* PAO1 virulence. PLoS One 2013; 8(1): e53441.
[http://dx.doi.org/10.1371/journal.pone.0053441] [PMID: 23320085]

[77]    Zhou L, Zheng H, Tang Y, Yu W, Gong Q. Eugenol inhibits quorum sensing at sub-inhibitory concentrations. Biotechnol Lett 2013; 35(4): 631-7.
[http://dx.doi.org/10.1007/s10529-012-1126-x] [PMID: 23264268]

[78]    Kalia M, Yadav VK, Singh PK, *et al.* Effect of cinnamon oil on quorum sensing-controlled virulence factors and biofilm formation in *Pseudomonas aeruginosa.* PLoS One 2015; 10(8): e0135495.
[http://dx.doi.org/10.1371/journal.pone.0135495] [PMID: 26263486]

[79]    Sheng JY, Chen TT, Tan XJ, Chen T, Jia AQ. The quorum-sensing inhibiting effects of stilbenoids and their potential structure-activity relationship. Bioorg Med Chem Lett 2015; 25(22): 5217-20.
[http://dx.doi.org/10.1016/j.bmcl.2015.09.064] [PMID: 26453007]

[80]    Banerjee M, Moulick S, Bhattacharya KK, Parai D, Chattopadhyay S, Mukherjee SK. Attenuation of *Pseudomonas aeruginosa* quorum sensing, virulence and biofilm formation by extracts of *Andrographis paniculata.* Microb Pathog 2017; 113: 85-93.
[http://dx.doi.org/10.1016/j.micpath.2017.10.023] [PMID: 29042302]

[81]    Reen FJ, Gutiérrez-Barranquero JA, Parages ML, O Gara F. Coumarin: a novel player in microbial quorum sensing and biofilm formation inhibition. Appl Microbiol Biotechnol 2018; 102(5): 2063-73.
[http://dx.doi.org/10.1007/s00253-018-8787-x] [PMID: 29392389]

[82]    Zhang D, Gan RY, Zhang JR, *et al.* Antivirulence properties and related mechanisms of spice essential oils: A comprehensive review. Compr Rev Food Sci Food Saf 2020; 19(3): 1018-55.
[http://dx.doi.org/10.1111/1541-4337.12549] [PMID: 33331691]

[83]    Borges A, Serra S, Cristina Abreu A, Saavedra MJ, Salgado A, Simões M. Evaluation of the effects of selected phytochemicals on quorum sensing inhibition and *in vitro* cytotoxicity. Biofouling 2014; 30(2): 183-95.
[http://dx.doi.org/10.1080/08927014.2013.852542] [PMID: 24344870]

[84]    Teasdale ME, Donovan KA, Forschner-Dancause SR, Rowley DC. Gram-positive marine bacteria as a potential resource for the discovery of quorum sensing inhibitors. Mar Biotechnol (NY) 2011; 13(4): 722-32.
[http://dx.doi.org/10.1007/s10126-010-9334-7] [PMID: 21152942]

[85]    Teasdale ME, Liu J, Wallace J, Akhlaghi F, Rowley DC. Secondary metabolites produced by the marine bacterium *Halobacillus salinus* that inhibit quorum sensing-controlled phenotypes in gram-negative bacteria. Appl Environ Microbiol 2009; 75(3): 567-72.
[http://dx.doi.org/10.1128/AEM.00632-08] [PMID: 19060172]

[86]    Tommonaro G, Abbamondi GR, Iodice C, Tait K, De Rosa S. Diketopiperazines produced by the halophilic archaeon, *Haloterrigena hispanica*, activate AHL bioreporters. Microb Ecol 2012; 63(3): 490-5.
[http://dx.doi.org/10.1007/s00248-011-9980-y] [PMID: 22109096]

[87]    Abed RM, Dobretsov S, Al-Fori M, Gunasekera SP, Sudesh K, Paul VJ. Quorum-sensing inhibitory compounds from extremophilic microorganisms isolated from a hypersaline cyanobacterial mat. J Ind Microbiol Biotechnol 2013; 40(7): 759-72.
[http://dx.doi.org/10.1007/s10295-013-1276-4] [PMID: 23645384]

[88]    Novick RP. Autoinduction and signal transduction in the regulation of staphylococcal virulence. Mol Microbiol 2003; 48(6): 1429-49.
[http://dx.doi.org/10.1046/j.1365-2958.2003.03526.x] [PMID: 12791129]

[89]    Borges A, Simões M. Quorum sensing inhibition by marine bacteria. Mar Drugs 2019; 17(7): 427.

[http://dx.doi.org/10.3390/md17070427] [PMID: 31340463]

[90]   Padmavathi AR, Abinaya B, Pandian SK. Phenol, 2,4-bis(1,1-dimethylethyl) of marine bacterial origin inhibits quorum sensing mediated biofilm formation in the uropathogen *Serratia marcescens.* Biofouling 2014; 30(9): 1111-22.
[http://dx.doi.org/10.1080/08927014.2014.972386] [PMID: 25377484]

[91]   de Carvalho MP, Abraham WR. Antimicrobial and biofilm inhibiting diketopiperazines. Curr Med Chem 2012; 19(21): 3564-77.
[http://dx.doi.org/10.2174/092986712801323243] [PMID: 22709011]

[92]   Tang K, Su Y, Brackman G, *et al.* MomL, a novel marine-derived N-acyl homoserine lactonase from *Muricauda olearia.* Appl Environ Microbiol 2015; 81(2): 774-82.
[http://dx.doi.org/10.1128/AEM.02805-14] [PMID: 25398866]

[93]   Hasan S, Ansari MI, Ahmad A, Mishra M. Major bioactive metabolites from marine fungi: A Review. Bioinformation 2015; 11(4): 176-81.
[http://dx.doi.org/10.6026/97320630011176] [PMID: 26124556]

[94]   Zhang M, Wang M, Zhu X, Yu W, Gong Q. Equisetin as potential quorum sensing inhibitor of *Pseudomonas aeruginosa.* Biotechnol Lett 2018; 40(5): 865-70.
[http://dx.doi.org/10.1007/s10529-018-2527-2] [PMID: 29502217]

[95]   Li X, Jeong JH, Lee KT, *et al.* Gamma-pyrone derivatives, kojic acid methyl ethers from a marine-derived fungus *Alternaria* sp. Arch Pharm Res 2003; 26: 532-4.
[http://dx.doi.org/10.1007/BF02976876] [PMID: 12934644]

[96]   Kong FD, Zhou LM, Ma QY, *et al.* Metabolites with Gram-negative bacteria quorum sensing inhibitory activity from the marine animal endogenic fungus *Penicillium* sp. SCS-KFD08. Arch Pharm Res 2017; 40(1): 25-31.
[http://dx.doi.org/10.1007/s12272-016-0844-3] [PMID: 27709333]

[97]   Miller MB, Bassler BL. Quorum sensing in bacteria. Annu Rev Microbiol 2001; 55: 165-99.
[http://dx.doi.org/10.1146/annurev.micro.55.1.165] [PMID: 11544353]

[98]   Paczkowski JE, Mukherjee S, McCready AR, *et al.* Flavonoids suppress *Pseudomonas aeruginosa* virulence through allosteric inhibition of quorum-sensing receptors. J Biol Chem 2017; 292(10): 4064-76.
[http://dx.doi.org/10.1074/jbc.M116.770552] [PMID: 28119451]

[99]   Weng LX, Yang YX, Zhang YQ, Wang LH. A new synthetic ligand that activates QscR and blocks antibiotic-tolerant biofilm formation in *Pseudomonas aeruginosa.* Appl Microbiol Biotechnol 2014; 98(6): 2565-72.
[http://dx.doi.org/10.1007/s00253-013-5420-x] [PMID: 24327212]

[100]  Capilato JN, Philippi SV, Reardon T, *et al.* Development of a novel series of non-natural triaryl agonists and antagonists of the *Pseudomonas aeruginosa* LasR quorum sensing receptor. Bioorg Med Chem 2017; 25(1): 153-65.
[http://dx.doi.org/10.1016/j.bmc.2016.10.021] [PMID: 27825554]

[101]  Geske GD, O'Neill JC, Miller DM, Mattmann ME, Blackwell HE. Modulation of bacterial quorum sensing with synthetic ligands: systematic evaluation of N-acylated homoserine lactones in multiple species and new insights into their mechanisms of action. J Am Chem Soc 2007; 129(44): 13613-25.
[http://dx.doi.org/10.1021/ja074135h] [PMID: 17927181]

[102]  Yadav MK, Park SW, Chae SW, Song JJ. Sinefungin, a natural nucleoside analogue of S-adenosylmethionine, inhibits Streptococcus pneumoniae biofilm growth. BioMed Res Int 2014; 2014: 156987.
[http://dx.doi.org/10.1155/2014/156987] [PMID: 25050323]

[103]  Hentzer M, Givskov M. Pharmacological inhibition of quorum sensing for the treatment of chronic bacterial infections. J Clin Invest 2003; 112(9): 1300-7.

[http://dx.doi.org/10.1172/JCI20074] [PMID: 14597754]

[104] Chan KG, Liu YC, Chang CY. Inhibiting N-acyl-homoserine lactone synthesis and quenching *Pseudomonas* quinolone quorum sensing to attenuate virulence. Front Microbiol 2015; 6: 1173.
[http://dx.doi.org/10.3389/fmicb.2015.01173] [PMID: 26539190]

[105] Surolia N, Surolia A. Triclosan offers protection against blood stages of malaria by inhibiting enoyl-ACP reductase of *Plasmodium falciparum*. Nat Med 2001; 7(2): 167-73.
[http://dx.doi.org/10.1038/84612] [PMID: 11175846]

[106] Copitch JL, Whitehead RN, Webber MA. Prevalence of decreased susceptibility to triclosan in *Salmonella enterica* isolates from animals and humans and association with multiple drug resistance. Int J Antimicrob Agents 2010; 36(3): 247-51.
[http://dx.doi.org/10.1016/j.ijantimicag.2010.04.012] [PMID: 20541914]

[107] Guendouze A, Plener L, Bzdrenga J, *et al.* Effect of quorum quenching lactonase in clinical isolates of *Pseudomonas aeruginosa* and comparison with quorum sensing inhibitors. Front Microbiol 2017; 8: 227.
[http://dx.doi.org/10.3389/fmicb.2017.00227] [PMID: 28261183]

[108] Chow JY, Yang Y, Tay SB, Chua KL, Yew WS. Disruption of biofilm formation by the human pathogen *Acinetobacter baumannii* using engineered quorum-quenching lactonases. Antimicrob Agents Chemother 2014; 58(3): 1802-5.
[http://dx.doi.org/10.1128/AAC.02410-13] [PMID: 24379199]

[109] Fan X, Liang M, Wang L, Chen R, Li H, Liu X. Aii810, a novel cold-adapted N-acylhomoserine lactonase discovered in a metagenome, can strongly attenuate *Pseudomonas aeruginosa* virulence factors and biofilm formation. Front Microbiol 2017; 8: 1950.
[http://dx.doi.org/10.3389/fmicb.2017.01950] [PMID: 29067011]

[110] Sakr MM, Aboshanab KM, Elkhatib WF, Yassien MA, Hassouna NA. Overexpressed recombinant quorum quenching lactonase reduces the virulence, motility and biofilm formation of multidrug-resistant *Pseudomonas aeruginosa* clinical isolates. Appl Microbiol Biotechnol 2018; 102(24): 10613-22.
[http://dx.doi.org/10.1007/s00253-018-9418-2] [PMID: 30310963]

[111] Mukherji R, Varshney NK, Panigrahi P, Suresh CG, Prabhune A. A new role for penicillin acylases: degradation of acyl homoserine lactone quorum sensing signals by *Kluyvera citrophila* penicillin G acylase. Enzyme Microb Technol 2014; 56: 1-7.
[http://dx.doi.org/10.1016/j.enzmictec.2013.12.010] [PMID: 24564895]

[112] Lee J, Lee I, Nam J, Hwang DS, Yeon KM, Kim J. Immobilization and stabilization of acylase on carboxylated polyaniline nanofibers for highly effective antifouling application via quorum quenching. ACS Appl Mater Interfaces 2017; 9(18): 15424-32.
[http://dx.doi.org/10.1021/acsami.7b01528] [PMID: 28414213]

[113] Bijtenhoorn P, Mayerhofer H, Müller-Dieckmann J, *et al.* A novel metagenomic short-chain dehydrogenase/reductase attenuates *Pseudomonas aeruginosa* biofilm formation and virulence on *Caenorhabditis elegans*. PLoS One 2011; 6(10): e26278.
[http://dx.doi.org/10.1371/journal.pone.0026278] [PMID: 22046268]

[114] Weiland-Bräuer N, Kisch MJ, Pinnow N, Liese A, Schmitz RA. Highly effective inhibition of biofilm formation by the first metagenome-derived AI-2 quenching enzyme. Front Microbiol 2016; 7: 1098.
[http://dx.doi.org/10.3389/fmicb.2016.01098] [PMID: 27468282]

[115] Pustelny C, Albers A, Büldt-Karentzopoulos K, *et al.* Dioxygenase-mediated quenching of quinolone-dependent quorum sensing in *Pseudomonas aeruginosa*. Chem Biol 2009; 16(12): 1259-67.
[http://dx.doi.org/10.1016/j.chembiol.2009.11.013] [PMID: 20064436]

[116] Hodgkinson JT, Galloway WR, Welch M, Spring DR. Microwave-assisted preparation of the quorum-sensing molecule 2-heptyl-3-hydroxy-4(1H)-quinolone and structurally related analogs. Nat Protoc 2012; 7(6): 1184-92.

[http://dx.doi.org/10.1038/nprot.2012.054] [PMID: 22635110]

[117] Han M, Gu J, Gao GF, Liu WJ. China in action: national strategies to combat against emerging infectious diseases. Sci China Life Sci 2017; 60(12): 1383-5.
[http://dx.doi.org/10.1007/s11427-017-9141-3] [PMID: 28887624]

[118] Brackman G, Cos P, Maes L, Nelis HJ, Coenye T. Quorum sensing inhibitors increase the susceptibility of bacterial biofilms to antibiotics *in vitro* and *in vivo*. Antimicrob Agents Chemother 2011; 55(6): 2655-61.
[http://dx.doi.org/10.1128/AAC.00045-11] [PMID: 21422204]

[119] Vadekeetil A, Saini H, Chhibber S, Harjai K. Exploiting the antivirulence efficacy of an ajoene-ciprofloxacin combination against *Pseudomonas aeruginosa* biofilm associated murine acute pyelonephritis. Biofouling 2016; 32(4): 371-82.
[http://dx.doi.org/10.1080/08927014.2015.1137289] [PMID: 26930141]

[120] Fong J, Yuan M, Jakobsen TH, *et al.* Disulfide bond-containing ajoene analogues as novel quorum sensing inhibitors of *Pseudomonas aeruginosa*. J Med Chem 2017; 60(1): 215-27.
[http://dx.doi.org/10.1021/acs.jmedchem.6b01025] [PMID: 27977197]

[121] García-Contreras R, Martínez-Vázquez M, Velázquez Guadarrama N, *et al.* Resistance to the quorum-quenching compounds brominated furanone C-30 and 5-fluorouracil in *Pseudomonas aeruginosa* clinical isolates. Pathog Dis 2013; 68(1): 8-11.
[http://dx.doi.org/10.1111/2049-632X.12039] [PMID: 23620228]

[122] Jakobsen TH, Bragason SK, Phipps RK, *et al.* Food as a source for quorum sensing inhibitors: iberin from horseradish revealed as a quorum sensing inhibitor of *Pseudomonas aeruginosa*. Appl Environ Microbiol 2012; 78(7): 2410-21.
[http://dx.doi.org/10.1128/AEM.05992-11] [PMID: 22286987]

[123] Bahari S, Zeighami H, Mirshahabi H, Roudashti S, Haghi F. Inhibition of *Pseudomonas aeruginosa* quorum sensing by subinhibitory concentrations of curcumin with gentamicin and azithromycin. J Glob Antimicrob Resist 2017; 10: 21-8.
[http://dx.doi.org/10.1016/j.jgar.2017.03.006] [PMID: 28591665]

[124] Chu C, Deng J, Man Y, Qu Y. Green tea extracts epigallocatechin-3-gallate for different treatments. BioMed Res Int 2017; 2017: 5615647.
[http://dx.doi.org/10.1155/2017/5615647] [PMID: 28884125]

[125] Inoue Y, Togashi N, Hamashima H. Farnesol-induced disruption of the *Staphylococcus aureus* cytoplasmic membrane. Biol Pharm Bull 2016; 39(5): 653-6.
[http://dx.doi.org/10.1248/bpb.b15-00416] [PMID: 27150138]

[126] Shao C, Shang W, Yang Z, *et al.* LuxS-dependent AI-2 regulates versatile functions in *Enterococcus faecalis* V583. J Proteome Res 2012; 11(9): 4465-75.
[http://dx.doi.org/10.1021/pr3002244] [PMID: 22856334]

[127] Anderson JK, Huang JY, Wreden C, *et al.* Chemorepulsion from the quorum signal autoinducer-2 promotes *Helicobacter pylori* biofilm dispersal. MBio 2015; 6(4): e00379.
[http://dx.doi.org/10.1128/mBio.00379-15] [PMID: 26152582]

[128] Thompson JA, Oliveira RA, Djukovic A, Ubeda C, Xavier KB. Manipulation of the quorum sensing signal AI-2 affects the antibiotic-treated gut microbiota. Cell Rep 2015; 10(11): 1861-71.
[http://dx.doi.org/10.1016/j.celrep.2015.02.049] [PMID: 25801025]

[129] Park H, Lee K, Yeo S, Shin H, Holzapfel W. Autoinducer-2 signalling in probiotics: a mechanism of gut microbiota modulation. Proceedings of the 2016 11th International Pipeline Conference. 56.

[130] Krzyżek P. Challenges and limitations of anti-quorum sensing therapies. Front Microbiol 2019; 10: 2473.
[http://dx.doi.org/10.3389/fmicb.2019.02473] [PMID: 31736912]

# CHAPTER 5

# Nitrogen and Oxygen-based Heterocycles as Potential Anti-Infective Agents

**Shaik Baji Baba[2], Naresh Kumar Katari[1,2,*] and Rambabu Gundla[1]**

[1] *Department of Chemistry, School of Science, GITAM Deemed to be University, Hyderabad, Telangana-502329, India*

[2] *School of Chemistry & Physics, College of Agriculture, Engineering & Science, Westville Campus, University of KwaZulu-Natal, P Bag X 54001, Durban-4000, South Africa*

**Abstract:** The success of Anti-infective agents (AIAs) is determined by the interaction between a drug and the binding sites. Significant contributions have been made to the synthetic and dynamic relationship between drugs and pharmacodynamics for the past few years. In general, AIAs include antibacterial, antiviral, antifungal, and antimicrobial agents, *etc.* The clinical benefit of using anti-infecting agents significantly impacts bloodstream infections with central venous catheters (CVCs), pregnancy, and lactation. Recent reports suggest income from AIGs formed 30.1% of the total income of hospitality management. However, many more technical difficulties remain, such as acquiring biologically relevant chemical diversity and achieving activity across diverse pathogens, including highly challenging Gram-negative pathogens with safe drugs. This chapter reviewed 1,2,4-triazoles, isatin, and coumarin-based anti-infective agent developments from the past five years and their biological studies against the various bacterial strains based on new challenges on viral and bacterial infections and viruses. SAR studies also discussed the importance of hybrids and substitutions in biology. We believe that this chapter helps future researchers to develop the most effective and less toxic anti-infective agents.

**Keywords:** Anti-infective agents, Coumarin, Isatin, Toxicity, Triazole.

## INTRODUCTION

Viruses include a large group of pathogens, which are the main ones responsible for producing different infectious diseases. More than 40% of the deaths worldwide are associated with various infectious diseases. From the past few dec-

* **Corresponding author Naresh Kumar Katari:** Department of Chemistry, School of Science, GITAM Deemed to be University, Hyderabad, Telangana, INDIA; & School of Chemistry & Physics, College of Agriculture, Engineering & Science, Westville Campus, University of KwaZulu-Natal, Durban, South Africa;
E-mail: dr.n.k.katari@gmail.com

**Parvesh Singh, Vipan Kumar & Rajshekhar Karpoormath (Eds.)**
**All rights reserved-© 2021 Bentham Science Publishers**

ades, the development of antiviral agents has played a pivotal role in the research. In the past 50 years, antiviral drugs directly targeted viral proteins and inhibited viral activity, showing better activity [1]. The world is facing different dangerous viruses such as Ebola, Spanish flu, cholera, *etc.* In 2019-2020, we fought with the most destructive virus, COVID-19 [2]. While developed nations were locked down and quarantined, they have also been struggling to establish a new class of antiviral drugs to kill the new type of Coronavirus. For the past few years, infectious diseases have been the leading cause of death worldwide [3]. In the 1940s, penicillin was introduced as an antibacterial agent from natural products. Natural and synthetic antibiotics have significant effects on human health. However, the treatment of viral and bacterial infections is a challenge because of a growing number of viruses and bacteria, which are multidrug-resistant microbial pathogens [4]. Many AIAs have been available in the market for the past few decades, but the need to develop a new class of drugs is required to minimise the side effects and toxicity. Reports from WHO indicate that diseases like pneumonia, an acquired immunodeficiency syndrome (AIDS), chronic liver disease, chronic obstructive lung disease, and neoplastic diseases like stomach cancers, cervical cancers, and liver cancers are the primary cause of human death worldwide. The severity of infectious diseases causes deaths every year due to AIDS (2.5 million), tuberculosis (1.8 million), and other diseases (more than one million due to malaria, dengue, and chikungunya) as per WHO reports [5]. The *Staphylococci, Pseudomonas aeruginosa*, and *Enterococci* are significant contributors of nosocomial type infections, which have also increased over the past few years. This infection is also known as hospital-acquired infection and is mainly transmitted *via* healthcare workers, hospital devices, and patients [6].

Antibiotics are the second most needed category of medication used in medical treatment. The mechanism of antibiotics includes bactericidal (bacteria killers) or bacteriostatic (inhibits microorganism multiplication). Most commonly known active bactericidal agents including penicillins, cephalosporins, and aminoglycosides such as neomycin, kanamycin, gentamicin, tobramycin, streptomycin, amikacin, and a few other bactericides are colistin, vancomycin, bacitracin, and polymyxin B. Bacteriostatic agents are clindamycin, sulphonamides, lincomycin, chloramphenicol, trimethoprim, erythromycin, and tetracyclines [7]. At present, inappropriate antibiotic usage and antibiotic resistance are major global issues because of a direct relation between antibiotics and antibiotic resistance developments. More than 85% of *Staphylococcus aureus* strains are resistant to penicillin and $\beta$-lactams in USA hospitals. Antimicrobial agents destroy the microorganism's structural parts or performed by interfering in microbial biosynthetic functions. Infective agents like chloramphenicol, tetracyclines, lincomycin, streptomycin, *etc.*, damage the protein synthesis and affect ribosomal subunits.

In 1963, Idoxuridine was the first antiviral drug introduced on the market. After that, nearly 95 antiviral drugs were approved in the past 50 years. Several types of antiviral drugs are developed for medical use to save human beings from viruses.

From 1993 to 2019, more than 110 antiviral drugs have been approved to treat nine different human viral infectious diseases. Few are under clinical trial phases, and thousands of antiviral agents and inhibitors are reported by multiple researchers globally [8]. The approved antiviral drugs are mainly characterised into thirteen functional groups to treat nine human viral infection diseases, shown in Table **1**.

**Table 1. Characterization of approving antiviral functional groups for nine human infectious viral diseases [8].**

| S. No | Viral Infection | Antiviral Agents/Class |
|---|---|---|
| 1 | Human immunodeficiency virus (HIV) | Protease inhibitors, integrase inhibitors, nucleoside reverse transcriptase inhibitors, acyclic nucleoside phosphonate analogues |
| 2 | Hepatitis B virus | Lamivudine, interferons, nucleoside analogues, *etc.* |
| 3 | Hepatitis C virus | Ribavirin, NS3/4A protease inhibitors, NS5A inhibitors, NS5B polymerase inhibitors |
| 4 | Herpesvirus infections | 5-substituted 2'-deoxyuridine analogues, pyrophosphate analogues, acyclic guanosine analogues |
| 5 | Influenza virus | Ribavirin, RNA polymerase inhibitors, and neuraminidase inhibitors, matrix two protein inhibitors |
| 6 | Human cytomegalovirus infections | Acyclic guanosine analogues, pyrophosphate analogues, and oligonucleotides |
| 7 | Varicella-zoster virus infections | Acyclic guanosine analogues, 5-substituted 2'-deoxyuridine analogues, and antibodies |
| 8 | Respiratory syncytial virus infections | Ribavirin and antibodies |
| 9 | Human papillomavirus | Imiquimod, podofilox and sinecatechins |

More effective antiviral drugs/vaccines to treat against emerging viruses such as the Ebola virus, Coronavirus, *etc.*, are not available in the present market. In the antiviral drug development journey, most of the approved antiviral agents are chemically synthesised hybrids. However, natural products play a prominent role in developing antivirals by providing insights into chemical compound synthesis for antiviral drugs [9]. Based on their broad spectrum, antiviral agents kill and inhibit the reproduction of viruses.

This chapter highlights the recent developments of 1,2,4-triazoles, isatin, and coumarin-based anti-infective agents such as antiviral and antibacterial agents based on their applications in medicinal chemistry against viral and bacterial strains. Many research studies have been reported from the past few years. All results indicate that nitrogen and oxygen-containing heterocyclics like isatin and triazole derivatives and coumarin-containing agents are more potential anti-infecting agents for future drug developments. Structure-activity relationship (SAR) studies also reveal the significant interaction between the binding site and selected moiety.

## 1,2,4-TRIAZOLES

In the present world, many infectious diseases are being identified. Research is being undertaken rapidly to overcome viral infections. Isoniazid, Rifampicin, Ethambutol, and Pyrazinamide have been mainly used to treat different conditions for the past 70 years, and still, they are playing a significant role mainly in tuberculosis (TB). The mechanism of action (MOA) contains several effects on lipids, proteins, glycolysis, nucleic acid synthesis, *etc* [10]. At the same time, these have many adverse effects, such as hepatitis, peripheral neuropathy, allergic reactions, and drug reactions [11, 12]. Due to its long-term action potential, isoniazid is the most common bacterial strain resistance because of these properties. There is an emerging area to introduce novel isoniazid derivatives.

1,2,4-Triazoles turn into the essential pharmacophore because of their significant interactions with biological receptors such as high affinity, rigidity, solubility, and hydrogen bonding. These are common integral parts in a variety of drugs that are available in the clinical treatment, such as fluconazole, itraconazole, posaconazole, voriconazole, ravuconazole for antifungal treatment, estazolam, alprazolam for anxiolytic effects, anticonvulsant and hypnotic effects, etizolam as an anxiolytic and skeletal muscle relaxant, rizatriptan for antimigraine activity, trapidil for antiplatelet activity, trazodone for antidepressant activity, anastrozole for anticancer activity, letrozole for aromatase inhibition, ribavirin for antiviral activity and loreclezole for anticonvulsant activity (Fig. **1**) [13]. For the past few decades, researchers have been developing novel triazole derivatives with a broad spectrum of activity, significant impact with less toxicity to fight against various bacterial and viral pathogens. Triazole compounds showed antifungal activity by inhibiting the cytochrome P450-dependent enzyme activity. The lanosterol 14$\alpha$-demethylase (CYP51) is the foremost important enzyme in the ergosterol biosynthesis of fungi [14, 15].

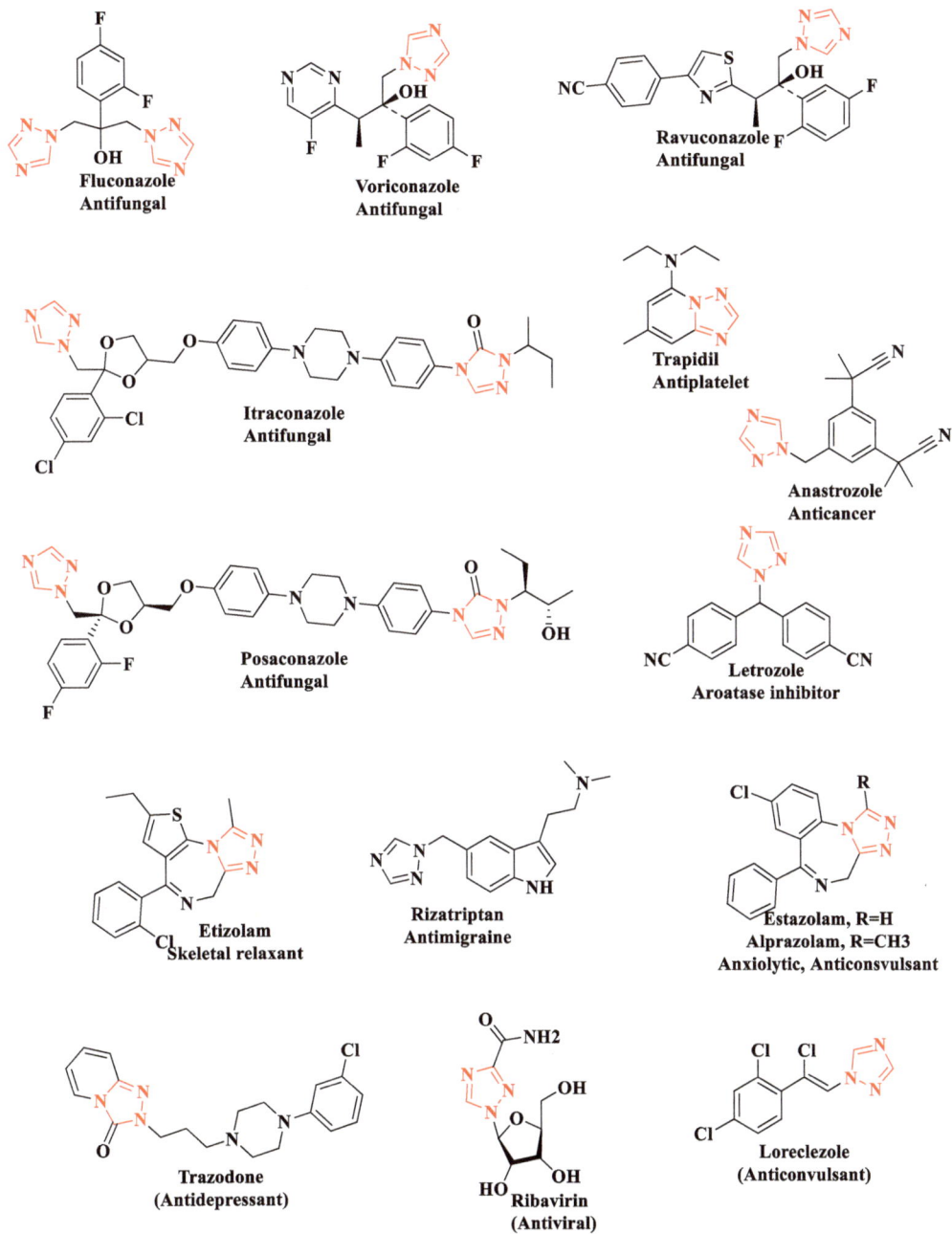

**Fig. (1).** 1,2,4-triazole scaffold in clinical applications [13].

## Antifungal Activity

Recent reports of *Wu et al.* designed, synthesised, and evaluated voriconazole derivatives **BB-1** (Fig. **2**) with amine substitutions or heterocycles as a side chain for antifungal activity *in vitro* and *in vivo* studies against various human pathogenic fungi [15]. From their results and docking studies, a compound containing morpholine moiety showed strong activity to inhibit the growth of the fungal pathogen (MIC$_{80}$: 0.0156 µg/mL). Many studies have reported the synthesis and antifungal evolution of the 1,2,4-triazole derivatives **B1-11** series shown in Fig. (**2**). Compound **BB-2** (Fig. **2**) has shown greater antifungal effect than fluconazole against *Candida albicans* (MIC$_{80}$: 0.0156 µg/mL) [16]. Compound **BB-3** (Fig. **2**) with trifluoromethyl substitution at R1 exhibits broad-spectrum antifungal activity (MIC$_{80}$: 0.00097µg/mL range) against the human pathogenic fungi (HPF) such as *C. Albicans, Candida parapsilosis, Candida tropicalis, Cryptococcus neoformans, Trichophyton rubrum, Fonsecaea compacta, and Microsporum gypseum*. It is shown to be 64-fold more effective than fluconazole and voriconazole reference drugs against *Aspergillus fumigatus* (MIC$_{80}$: 1 µg/mL) [17]. Compound **BB-6** (Fig. **2**) exhibits significant antifungal activity against the *C. Albicans* (MIC: 0.0625 µg/mL) [18]. Triazole moieties of compounds **BB-7, BB-8** (Fig. **2**) with heterocycle-benzene bioisosteric replacement reported good antifungal activity with great oral absorption. Fluconazole derivatives of **BB-9** (Fig. **2**) have shown high antifungal activity against the *C. Albicans, C. Neoformans, C. Parapsilosis,* and *Candida glabrata* (MIC$_{80}$: <0.125 µg/mL) [12]. For compound **BB-10** (Fig. **2**), SAR studies show that the greatest activity against the *C. Albicans* (MIC$_{80}$=0.0039 µg/mL) is achieved mainly with 2-Cl and 3-Cl substitutions [19]. Li *et al.* designed the isoxazole with triazole moiety of ravuconazole **BB-11** (Fig. **2**) **a-c** show greater activity than ravuconazole against various fungal species [20].

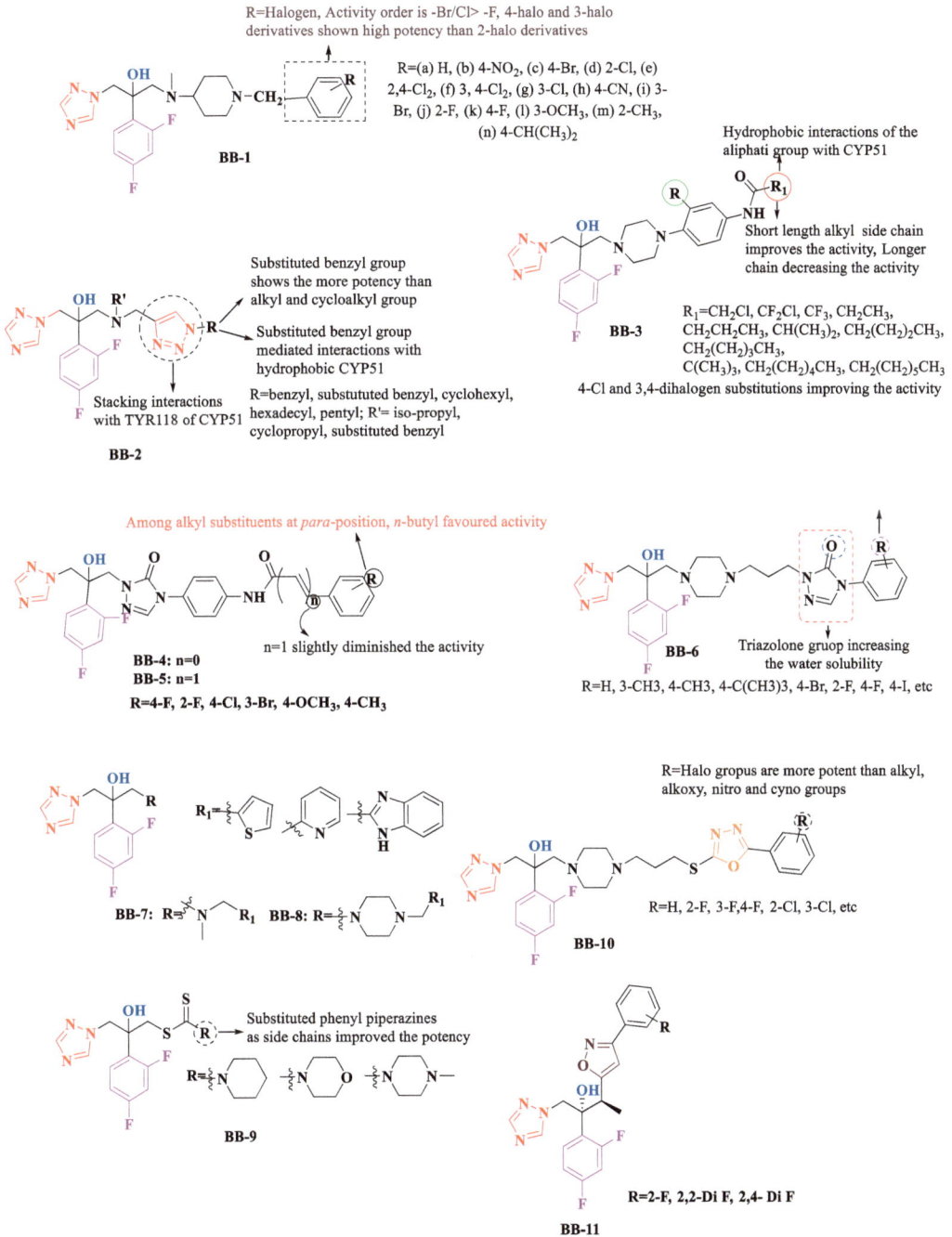

**Fig. (2).** SAR studies and antifungal activity of 1,2,4-triazole derivatives [15 - 20].

*Cao et al.* designed and synthesized the novel fused heterocycles linked triazoles and evaluated the SAR studies. SAR studies have shown that multi-halogenated indole derivatives of triazoles are exhibit a 4-fold increase in antifungal activity against the *C. Albicans, A. fumigatus*, and *C. krusei* [21]. Amongst all the compounds, **BB-12** (Fig. **3**) shows the most potent activity against the *Candida, Cryptococcus, Aspergillus* species. *Shrestha et al.* designed and synthesized a novel alkylated azole derivative **BB-13** (Fig. **3**) .Biological analysis results exhibit less cytotoxicity and high activity against *C. Albicans*, non-*Albicans Candida*, and *Aspergillus strains* [22]. *Zhang et al.* synthesized the novel hybrid carbazole-triazole moieties **BB-14** (Fig. **3**) and studied the antifungal activity against *C. Albicans, C. Tropicalis, C. Parapsilosis*, and *A. Fumigatus* [23].

Recently, *Lin et al.* reported the antifungal nature of novel myrtenal-based 4-methyl-1,2,4-triazole-thioethers **BB-15** (Fig. **3**) . The report reveals that many compounds have shown improved activity compared to myrtenal and indicates that the combination of 1,2,4-triazole-thioether with myrtenal benefits the antifungal activity. Few compounds showed high activity against the *P. piricola* when compared to azoxystrobin [24].

*Jin et al.* designed and synthesized the novel 1,2,4-triazole Schiff base **BB-16D** (Fig. **3**) derivatives which revealed biological activity against the fungal species. These Schiff bases $EC_{50}$=0.0087 g/L exhibit more antifungal activity than triadimefon $EC_{50}$: 0.0195 g/L against the *Gibberlla nicotiancola* and *Gibberlla saubinetii* [25]. A novel sulfonamide-1,2,4-triazoles, 1,3,4-thiadiazoles **BB-17** (Fig. **3**), and 1,3,4-oxadiazoles are potential antibacterial and antifungal agents [26] with few fungi like *A. niger, Trichoderma viride,* and *Aspergillus flavus*. The results showed that compared to bifonazole and ketoconazole commercial agents, it showed 10-60 times more activity and exhibited great antifungal activity structure.

*Tang et al.* Synthesizes the amide derivatives having 1,2,4-triazoles **BB-18** (Fig. **3**) . These results show the antifungal and antibacterial activity against at 50 mg/L with *Gibberella azeae, Fusarium oxysporum, Cytospora mandshurica, Pellicularia sasakii,* and *Phytophthora infestans* [27].

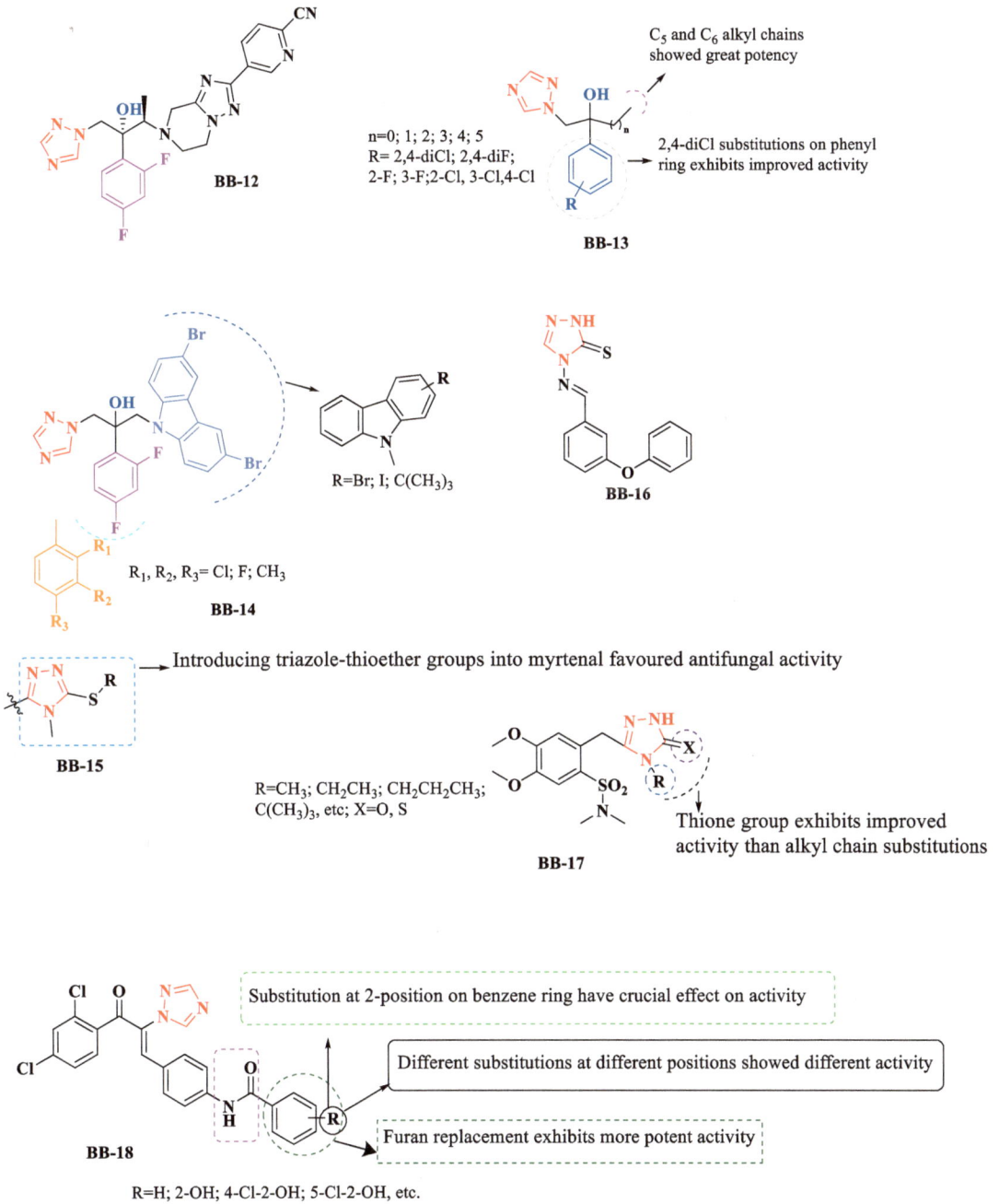

**Fig. (3).** 1,2,4-triazole derivatives as potential antifungal agents and SAR studies [21 - 27].

## Antibacterial Activity

Triazole derivatives have significant applications in antibacterial activity. Compared to chloramphenicol, clinafloxacin, and fluconazole, synthesised triazole contains clinafloxacin hybrids that show good antibacterial and fungal activity [28]. SAR study of compounds **B1a-g** (Fig. **4**) reveals excellent antibacterial and antifungal activity (MIC: 0.25 μg/mL) against *Staphylococcus aureus*. *Plech et al.* investigated the antibacterial activity of 1,2,4-triazol--ciprofloxacin hybrids **B2** (Fig. **4**) (MIC: 0.046 μM) against the pathogen panels, and it was found to have improved potency against the MRSA compared to reference samples of vancomycin and Ciprofloxacin [29]. For compound **B2** (Fig. **4**), SAR studies open that the C3 position in the phenyl group plays a pivotal role for high activity. The -OH group on the phenyl ring increases the activity, and the N-4 position in the alkyl chain impacts the activity.

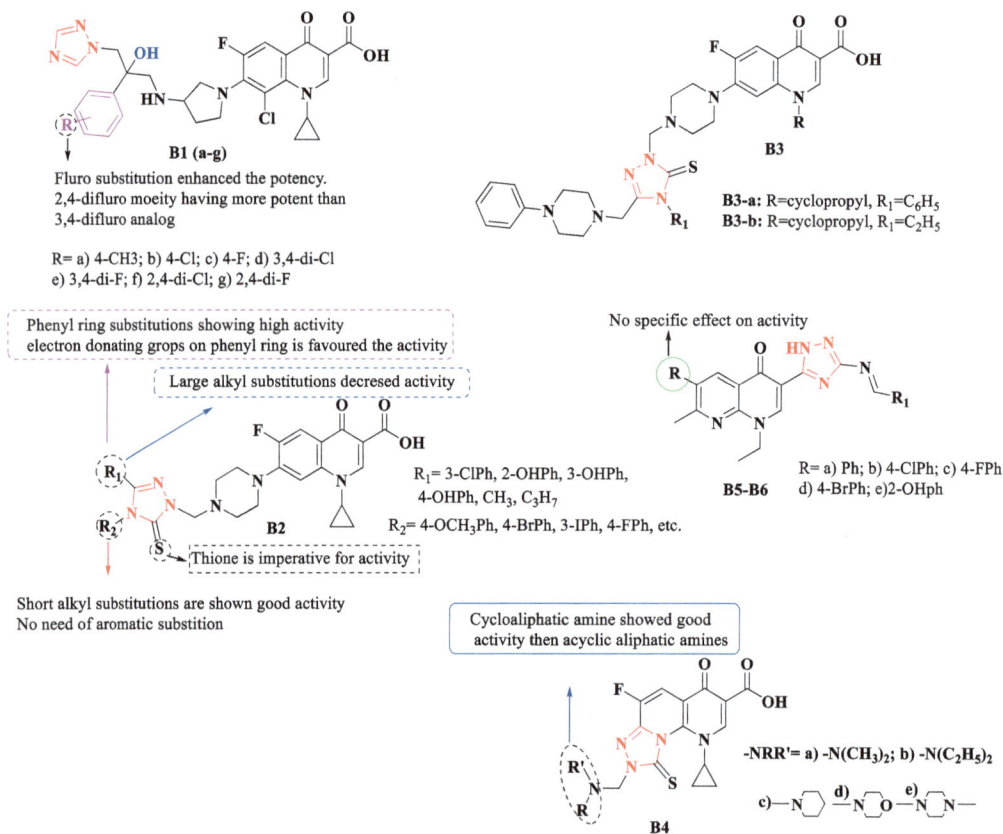

**Fig. (4).** 1,2,4-triazole based potent antibacterial agents and their SAR results [28 - 32].

Piperazine-triazole-quinolone hybrids **B3** (Fig. **4**) are shown to possess good antibacterial activity against the *Escherichia coli, Pseudomonas aeruginosa, Klebsiella pneumoniae, Acinetobacter haemolyticus, Enterococcus faecalis, Staphylococcus aureus,* in compounds **B3-a** (Fig. **4**) and **B3-b** (Fig. **4**) they exhibit more excellent activity MIC: 0.125 µg/mL [30]. *Gao et al.* designed and synthesised a novel [1, 2, 4]triazolo[3,4-h] [1, 8]naphthyridine-7-carboxylic acid derivatives **B4** (Fig. **4**), at the C8 position, it exhibits a significant antibacterial efficiency [31]. *Mohamed et al.* developed a triazole-naphthyridinone hybrids **B5** (Fig. **4**) and **B6** (Fig. **4**) and studied the antimicrobial activities against the *Gram-positive, Gram-negative* strains and **B5-a**, **B5-f**, **B5-g**, **B6-a**, and **B6-d** (Fig. **4**) shown outstanding activity against the *Bacillus subtilis* (MIC: 3.68 µM/mL) and also studied the **B5-c** and **B6-d** (Fig. **4**) antibacterial inhibitory efficiency against the *E. coli* DNA gyrase [32].

1,2,4-Triazolo with thiadiazine hybrid derivatives **B7** (Fig. **5**) screened for antibacterial activity against four different human pathogenic bacteria such as *E. coli, K. pneumonia, S. dysenteriae,* and *Shigella flexnei* at 100 µg/mL concentrations. In all compounds**B7-d** (Fig. **5**), the inhibitory zone exhibits the potential activity compared to standard neomycin and streptomycin, it showing good antibacterial inhibitory activity [33]. *Hashem et al.* designed a novel 1,2,4-triazolopyrimidines containing thiourea moieties **B8** (Fig. **5**). They performed the antibacterial activity analysis against the different bacteria like *E. coli, S. aureus, P. aeruginosa, B. subtilis,* and antimicrobial effectiveness against the *Geotrichum candidum, A. fumigatus, Syncephalastrum racemosum,* and *Aspergillus fumigatus* and all derivatives have shown remarkable efficacy against the bacteria and fungi [34]. 1,2,4-Triazolo[1,5-a]pyrimidines with thioether quinazoline group **B9** (Fig. **5**) influenced efficiency in the activity against the phytopathogenic bacteria in this compound **B9-a** (Fig. **5**) exhibited more activity against the *Xanthomonas oryzae pv. Oryzae* ($EC_{50}$: 7.2 µg/mL) than ($EC_{50}$: 89.8 µg/mL) of bismerthiazol studied by *Fan et al.* [35]. Triazolo-thiadiazole with thiouracil derivatives **B10(a-l)** (Fig. **5**) shown good antibacterial activity against the *Bacillus amyloliquefaciens, Bacillus subtilis,* and *Staphylococcus aureus* in that **B10-d** demonstrated inhibitory activity against *SecA* ATPase [36].

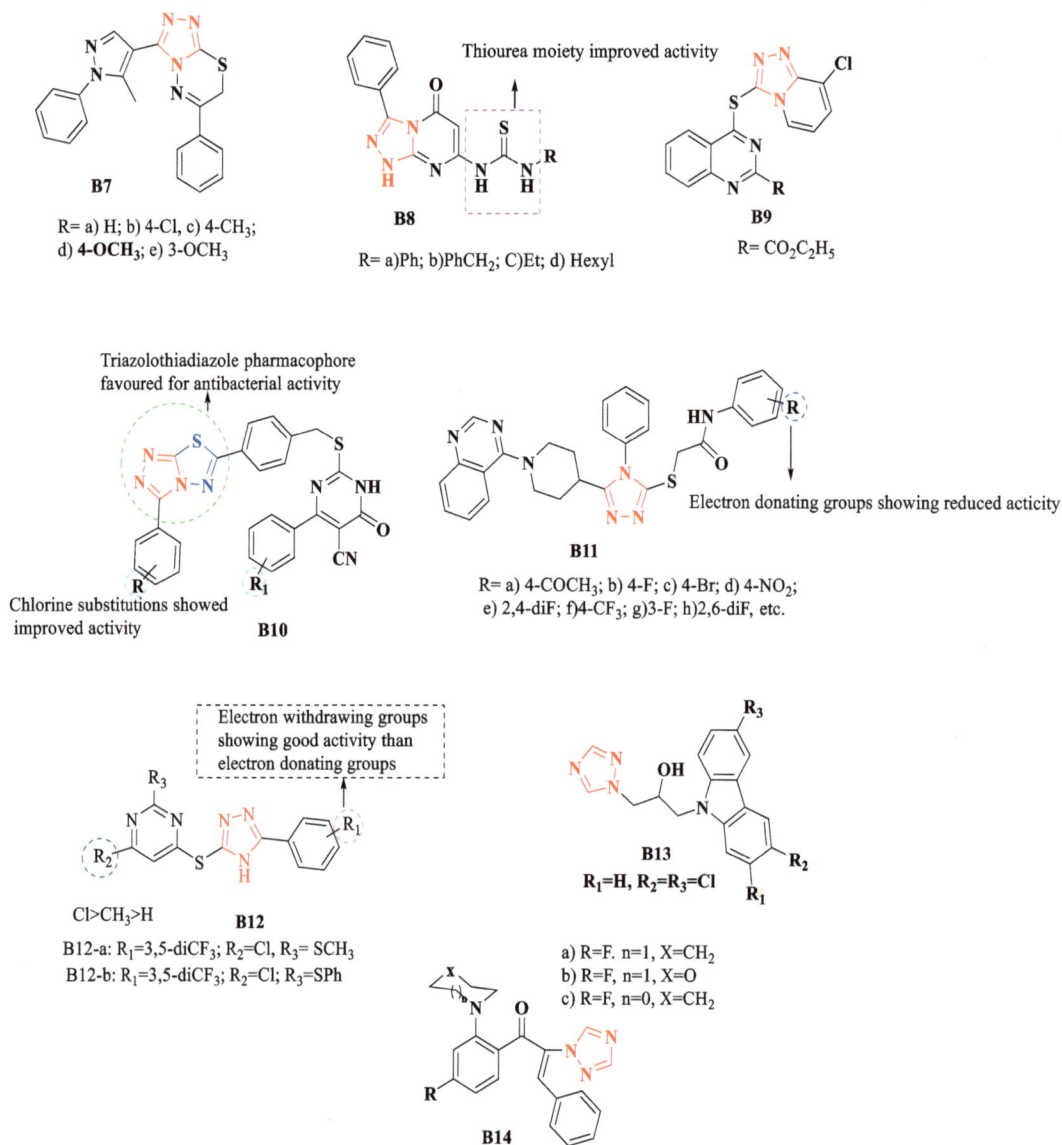

**B7**

R= a) H; b) 4-Cl, c) 4-CH$_3$;
d) **4-OCH$_3$**; e) 3-OCH$_3$

Thiourea moiety improved activity

**B8**

R= a)Ph; b)PhCH$_2$; C)Et; d) Hexyl

**B9**

R= CO$_2$C$_2$H$_5$

Triazolothiadiazole pharmacophore
favoured for antibacterial activity

Chlorine substitutions showed
improved activity **B10**

Electron donating groups showing reduced acticity

**B11**

R= a) 4-COCH$_3$; b) 4-F; c) 4-Br; d) 4-NO$_2$;
e) 2,4-diF; f)4-CF$_3$; g)3-F; h)2,6-diF, etc.

Electron withdrawing groups
showing good activity than
electron donating groups

Cl>CH$_3$>H **B12**

B12-a: R$_1$=3,5-diCF$_3$; R$_2$=Cl, R$_3$= SCH$_3$
B12-b: R$_1$=3,5-diCF$_3$; R$_2$=Cl; R$_3$=SPh

**B13**
R$_1$=H, R$_2$=R$_3$=Cl

a) R=F. n=1, X=CH$_2$
b) R=F, n=1, X=O
c) R=F, n=0, X=CH$_2$

**B14**

**Fig. (5).** 1,2,4-triazole based potent antibacterial hybrids and SAR study [33 - 40].

*Yang* and co-workers developed a novel 1,2,4-triazole containing the quinazolinyl-piperidinyl ring and N-(substituted phenyl) acetamide **B11** (Fig. **5**) functional substitutions with antibacterial and antimicrobial activities [37]. Among all these compounds, **B11-e**, **B11-g**, **B11-i**, **B11-l** (Fig. **5**) shown improved antibacterial activity compared to bismerthiazol against phytopathogenic bacterium *X. oryzae pv. Oryzae* ($EC_{50}$: 34.5 µg/mL).

*Cui et al.* synthesised triazole-pyrimidine analogues **B12** (Fig. **5**) and evaluated biological evolutions against S. *aureus* and *E. coli.* SAR studies showed strong electron-withdrawing group substitutions like 2,4-di-F, 3-F, 3-$NO_2$, 3-$COCH_3$, and 2-$NO_2$ on benzene rings exhibit improved activity [38]. *Zhang et al.* synthesised the isopropanol-conjugated carbazole triazoles **B13** (Fig. **5**) and screened the antibacterial property of these compounds against *E. faecalis, S. aureus*, and *E. coli.* This series of compound **B13-a** (MIC: 2 µg/mL) displayed improved potential activity against *E. faecalis* [39]. *Yin et al.* introduced the novel α-triazolyl chalcone derivatives **B14** (Fig. **5**) for their promising antimicrobial and antibacterial activity. They exhibited more significant activity (MIC: 3.8 µg/mL) against the MRSA than *chloromycin* [40].

## Antiviral Agents

Triazoles also have great applications in antibacterial potency. A recent study by *Goma et al.* synthesised the novel 1,2,4-triazole derivatives and screened biological evolution. Among all these compounds, compound **C1** (Fig. **6**) showed the most potent activity, decreasing the viral signs by 50-60% dose of 80 µM against the *herpes simplex virus-1* and exhibits more selectivity than acyclovir [41]. *Biswas et al.* synthesized the 4-aryl-6,7,8,9-tetrahydrobenzo [4, 5]thieno[3,2-e] [1, 2, 4]triazolo[4,3-a]pyrimidin-5(4H)-ones **C2** (Fig. **6**). They studied against the human enteroviruses such as *Coxsackievirus B1* (Cox B1), *Coxsackievirus B3* (Cox B3), *Poliovirus 3* (PV3), *Human Rhinovirus 14* (HRV14), *Human Rhinovirus 21* (HRV 21), and *Human Rhinovirus 71* (HRV 71). Results have shown that compound **C2** (Fig. **6**) shown good activity and that compound **C2** introduced broad spectral antiviral drugs [42]. *Zahabi et al.* synthesised some novel triazole-quinoxaline derivatives and evaluated these compounds as antiviral activity against the *hepatitis C* virus, *hepatitis B* virus, *Herpes simplex virus-1*, and *human cytomegalovirus* [43]. *In vitro* evaluation of these compounds indicated that pyridinyl containing triazole derivative **C3** (Fig. **6**) showed greater potential activity against *human cytomegalovirus* ($IC_{50}$: <0.05 µM) than the ganciclovir drug ($IC_{50}$: 0.59 µM). *Zaher* and co-workers designed and synthesised sixteen novel triazole derivatives **C4** (Fig. **6**) and screened for anti-middle east respiratory syndrome-related *Coronavirus* (MERS-CoV) activity *via* helicase inhibition and ATPase activity. Compounds **C4-a** and **C4-b** exhibit more potent MERS-CoV helicase inhibitors with ATPase ($IC_{50}$: 0.47 & 0.51 µmol/L) [44]. *Wang* and *co-workers* synthesised a set of novel acetamide substituted doravirine derivatives **C4** as potential HIV-1 non-nucleoside reverse-transcriptase inhibitors. The study reveals that the **C4** compound ($EC_{50}$: 54.8 nM) has shown good antiviral activity against HIV-1 and has a higher potency than lamivudine with $EC_{50}$: 12.8 µM reference sample [45].

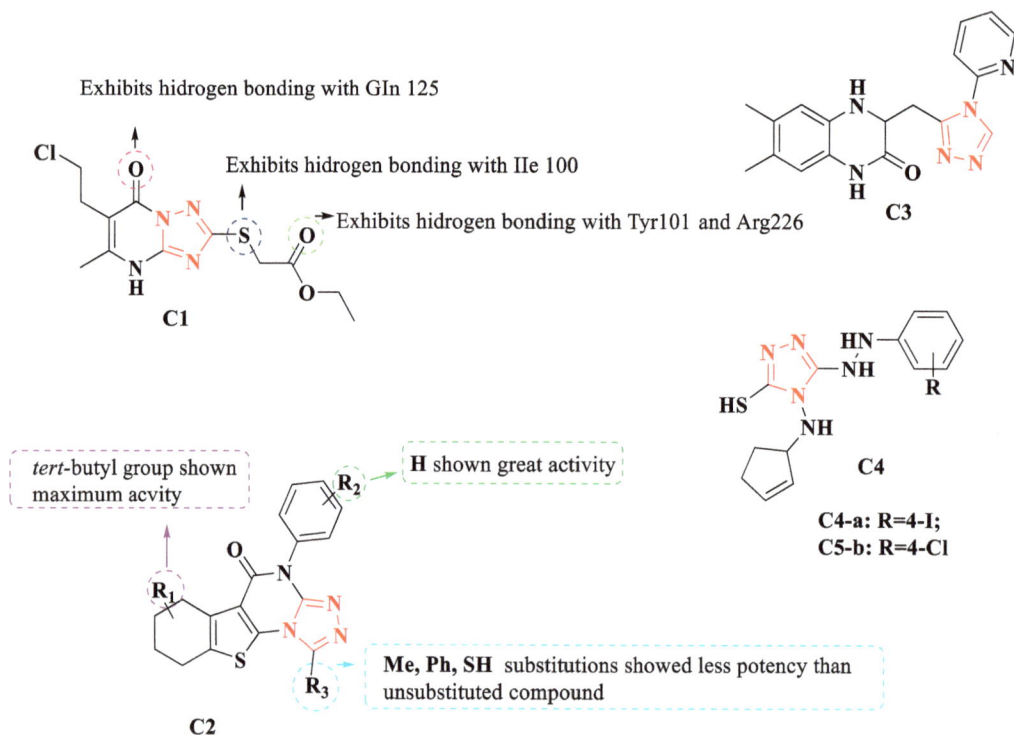

**Fig. (6).** 1,2,4-triazole based antiviral agents [41 - 45].

## ISATIN: (1*H*-INDOLE- 2,3-DIONE)

Isatin has excellent applications in drug development and has perfect pharmacological activity. Isatin is also branded as tribulin. It is one of the indole derivatives, and the molecular formula is $C_8H_5NO_2$. Heterocyclics with isatin exhibit great pharmacological activity such as antiviral, anticonvulsant, antitubercular, antimicrobial, anticancer, and many more applications in medicinal chemistry. Many researchers are working with the isatin pharmacophore by using the advantages of the first position, which has NH and $C_2$, $C_3$ carbonyl positions to help design various derivatives with greater biological activities. Isatin has a chemical structure containing the 6-membered carbon ring and 5-membered carbon ring with the nitrogen atom, which is more favourable for activity. Both aromatic rings are in the same plane. A few isatin ring-containing drugs which are on the market are shown in Fig. (7).

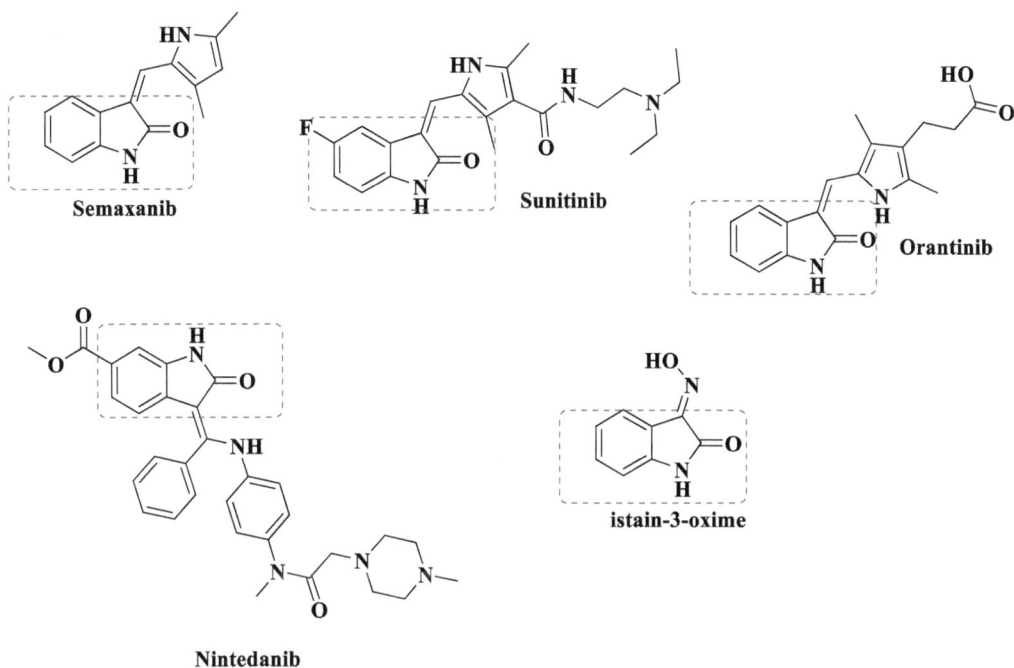

**Fig. (7).** Examples of isatin based marketed drugs.

## Antiviral Agents

In early 1952, *Chikungunya virus* disease was first found in Tanzania, and it is the most challenging viral infection, with the symptoms including fever, myalgia, nausea, body pains, and body rashes. Right now, there is no particular antiviral drug for the diagnosis and prevention of the Chikungunya virus. In 2016, Mishra and co-workers designed and synthesised the 1-[(2-methyl benzimidazole-1-yl)methyl]-2-oxo-indolin-3-ylidene]amino]thiourea **D1** (Fig. **8**) *via* hybridisation of an isatin derivative with 2-methyl benzimidazole. The synthesised derivatives are screened for biological activity and exhibited good antiviral activity against the *chikungunya* virus. The test results indicated that these compounds decreased the infection rate up to 76.03% [46]. *Nisha et al.* synthesised a Cu(I)Cl-promoted N-propargylated isatin-mannich adducts **D2** (Fig. **8**) and studied biological response against the *Trichomonas vaginalis*. Their analysis revealed that introducing the 4-aminoquinoline moiety shows improved activity, mainly with H and Cl substitutions exhibiting the more growth inhibition percentage rate, likely 92.15% and 100% [47]. *V. Kumar et al.* developed a 1H-1,2,3-triazole linked - lactam-isatin derivatives using click chemistry and screened against the *T. vaginalis* strains. The Compound **D3** (Fig. **8**) with phenyl substitution at N-1 of the lactam ring exhibited high activity (IC$_{50}$: 7.69 µM) and revealed a noncytotoxic nature. They also extended their work and synthesised the isatin uracil hybrids and evaluated the biological response against the *T. vaginalis*, **D4** (Fig. **8**) derivative with Cl substitution exhibits an improved antiviral activity profile (IC$_{50}$: 9.79 µg/mL) [48]. *Mohamed et al.* reported the 5-Fluoro-isatin thiosemicarbazone with methoxyphenyl, and different positions with methoxyphenyl are developed and evaluated the biological activity. Among all compounds, **D5** (Fig. **8**) exhibits the improved growth inhibition rate against the *Salmonella spp, including Salmonella enteritidis* and *Salmonella typhimurium,* and these derivatives are shown good DNA protection. Derivative **D6** (Fig. **8**) exhibits more DNA binding affinity [49].

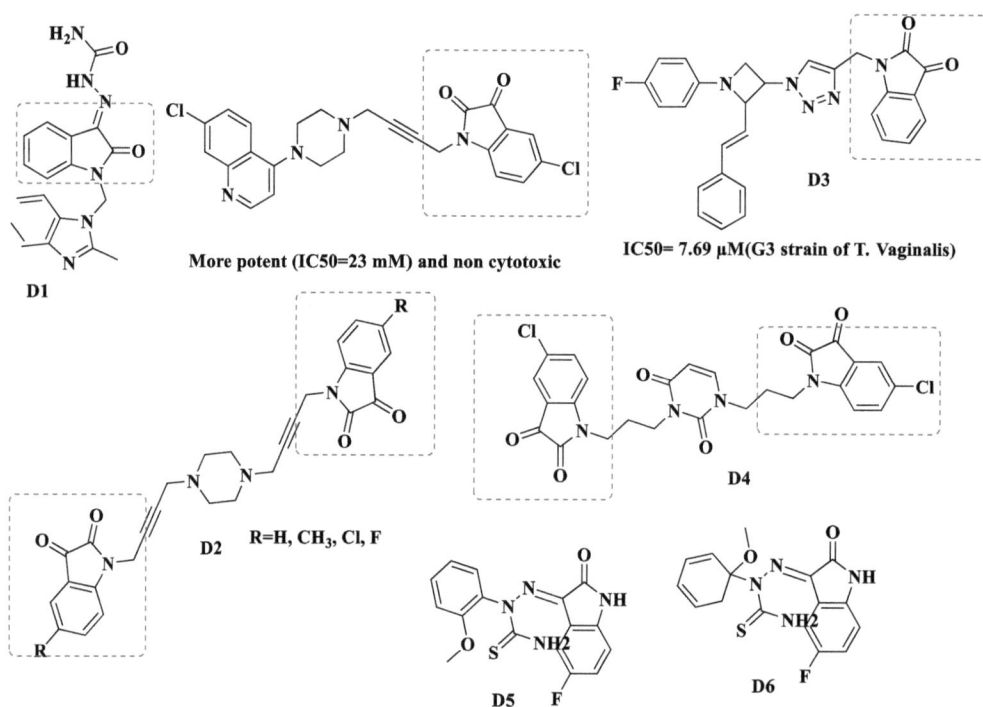

**Fig. (8).** Isatin-based most potential antiviral hybrids [46 - 49].

## Antibacterial Agents

*Bhagat* and co-workers designed and developed a new coumarin derivative with isatin compounds and evaluated the biological response against *Escherichia coli* and *Salmonella enterica*. **D7** (Fig. **9**) and **D8** (Fig. **9**) exhibited the most potent antibacterial activity among all compounds. Compound **D7** (MIC: 30 ug/mL) was active against the *Penicillium spp.,* and compound **D8** (Fig. **9**) was active against the *S. aureus* (MIC: 312 ug/mL). Compound **D8** docking studies revealed various interactions on the dihydrofolate reductase enzyme active sites [50]. Currently, novel isatin-indole hybrids are shown to possess the most promising antibacterial and antimicrobial activity. *Almutairi* and co-workers designed and synthesised new indole-isatin based hybrid derivatives and screened their biological evolution against the gram-negative bacteria such as *E. coli, P. aeruginosa, P Vulgaris, Klebsiella pneumonia,* and *Salmonella enteritidis* and gram-positive strains like *S. aureus, Methicillin-resistant S. aureus* (MRSA), *Enterococcus fecalis,* and *Bacillus subtilis* [51]. In this series, compounds **D9** (Fig. **9**) and **D10** (Fig. **9**) showed high potential activity against gram +ve and gram -ve bacteria.

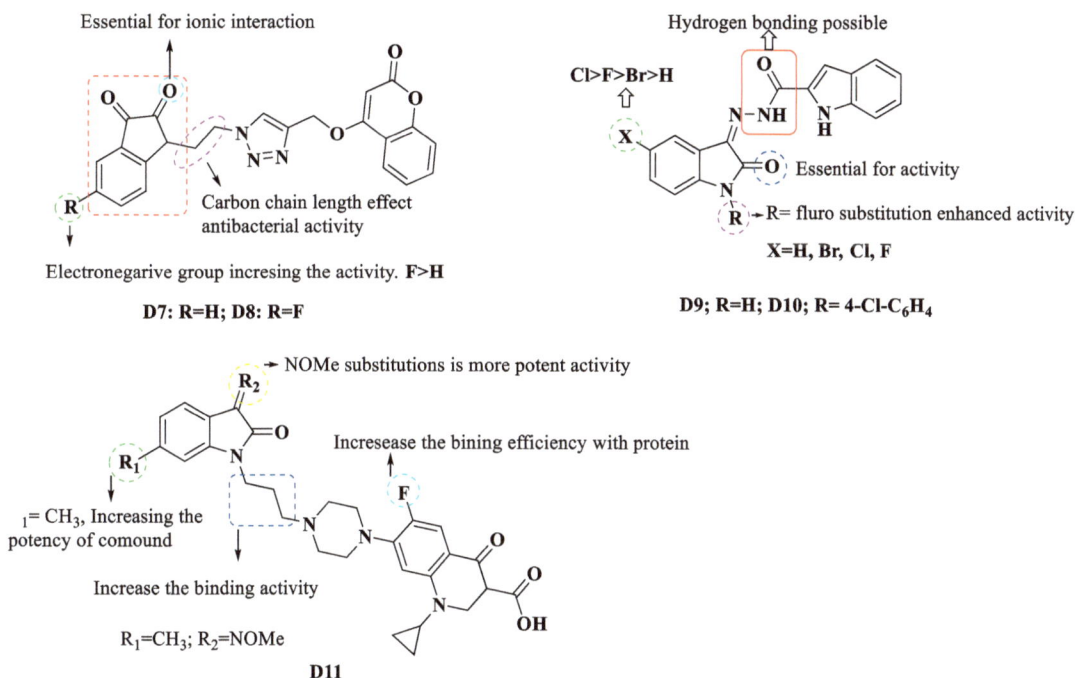

Fig. (9). Isatin derivatives as potential antibacterial agents and SAR study [50 - 52].

In 2018, *Wang* and co-workers designed and developed novel ciprofloxacin-isatin hybrids with propylene substitution hybrids and studied the antimicrobial and antibacterial activity against gram-positive and gram-negative bacterial strains. The compound **D11** (Fig. **9**) exhibits high potential activity against the bacterial strains [52].

Isatin-indole-coumarin hybrid structured molecules possess an excellent pharmacological property and exhibit a non-toxic nature. *Jin* and co-workers synthesised the isatin–1,2,3□triazole–coumarin hybrid derivatives **D12** (Fig. **10**) and studied the antibacterial activity against *E. coli* [53]. The SAR study revealed that the shorter alkyl link between the isatin and triazole, oxime at C3, and electron-donating groups at C5 positions in isatin are beneficial for antibacterial activity. From their developments, compound **D12-a, b** (MIC: 15 μg/ml) was active against the bacterial strain, and hybrid **D12-b** has been identified as the crucial scaffold in future research into novel antibacterial drugs as it possesses high activity. A class of Ciprofloxacin-containing isatin derivatives is evaluated as a potent antimicrobial and antibacterial activity against the bacterial strains by *Guo* [54]. Synthesised compounds exhibit good antibacterial and antimicrobial properties against gram-positive and gram-negative strains, including *S. epidermidis, Staphylococcus aureus, Enterococcus faecalis*, and *Enterococcus faecium*. Among all, **D13** (Fig. **10**) and **D14** (Fig. **10**) were exhibited the most potency from all the compounds.

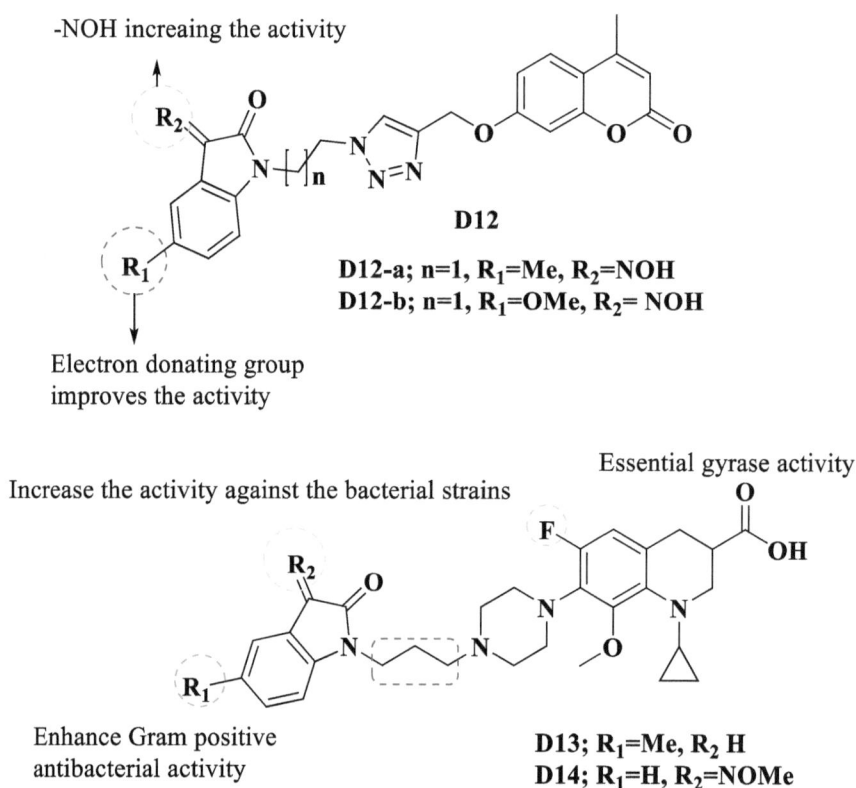

**Fig. (10).** Isatin-based antiviral agents [53, 54].

## Antitubercular Agents

*Gao et al.* design and developed moxifloxacin-acetyl-1,2,3-1H-triazolemethyene-isatin hybrids **D15** (Fig. **11**) and **D16** (Fig. **11**) *via* click chemistry evaluated anti-TB activity. Synthesised hybrids are exhibited for their biological property against the *Mycobacterium tuberculosis* strains. From their results, **D15** and **D16** (MIC: 0.12 µg/mL) showed the most potent activity compared to the moxifloxacin reference drug [55]. Furthermore, they also designed 20 novel derivatives of isatin-benzofuran-imine hybrids **D17** (Fig. **11**) and evaluated their anti-TB and antibacterial activity and cytotoxic nature. All synthesised hybrids have significantly shown *in vitro* anti-TB (MIC: 4.8 mg/mL) and antibacterial (MIC: 1 mg/mL) against the gram-positive and negative bacterial strains [56].

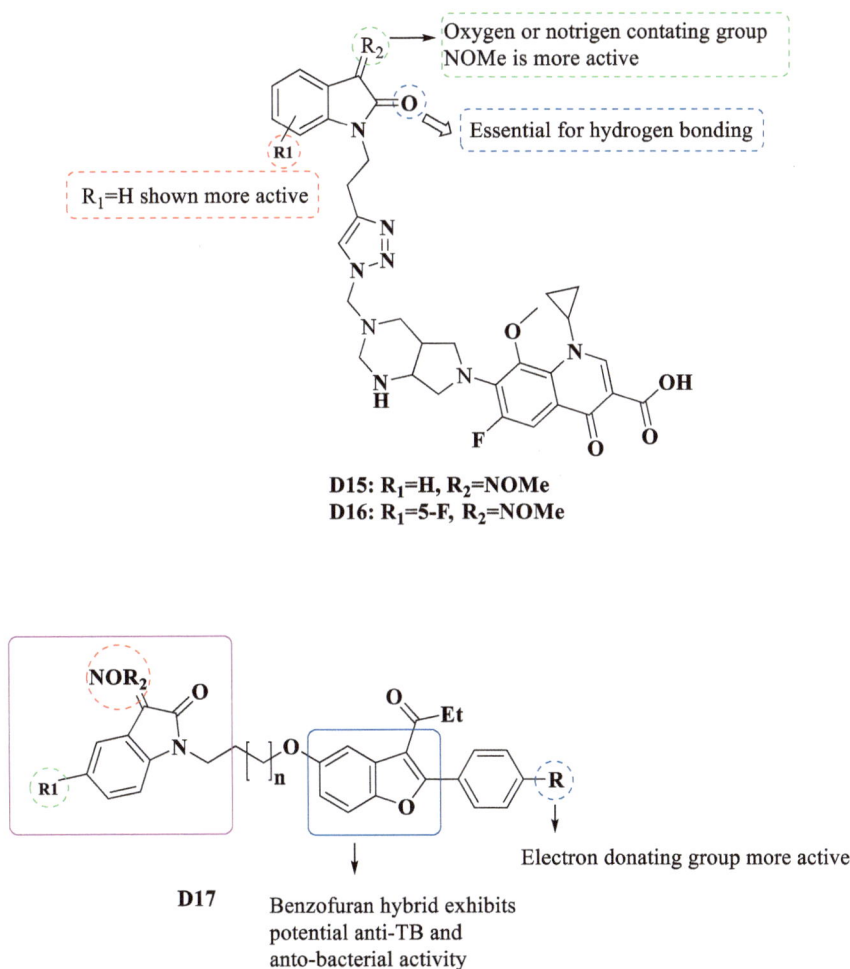

D15: R₁=H, R₂=NOMe
D16: R₁=5-F, R₂=NOMe

D17     Benzofuran hybrid exhibits
        potential anti-TB and
        anto-bacterial activity

**Fig. (11).** Isatin derivatives as a potential anti-TB agent and SAR study [55, 56].

## COUMARIN

Coumarin is a naturally occurring metabolite in various sources like plants, bacteria, fungi, oils and is also synthesised by chemical routes. In the past few years, coumarins have been isolated from different plants like *Umbelliferae*, *Rutaceae*, *etc.*, [57]. Based on its biological activities and pharmacological importance, coumarins have become a most encouraging and vital area for research in developing various antibacterial, antiviral, anticancer, anti TB, antimicrobial agents, *etc.* Numerous coumarin derivatives have been synthesised in the past few decades, and developed compounds exhibit great biological activities. SAR studies reveal the tremendous binding nature. Few synthetic coumarins with favourable pharmacophore groups at C3, C4, C7 positions are surprising with their biological activities. Various coumarin-based drugs have been developed in the past few decades and are shown in Fig. (**12**).

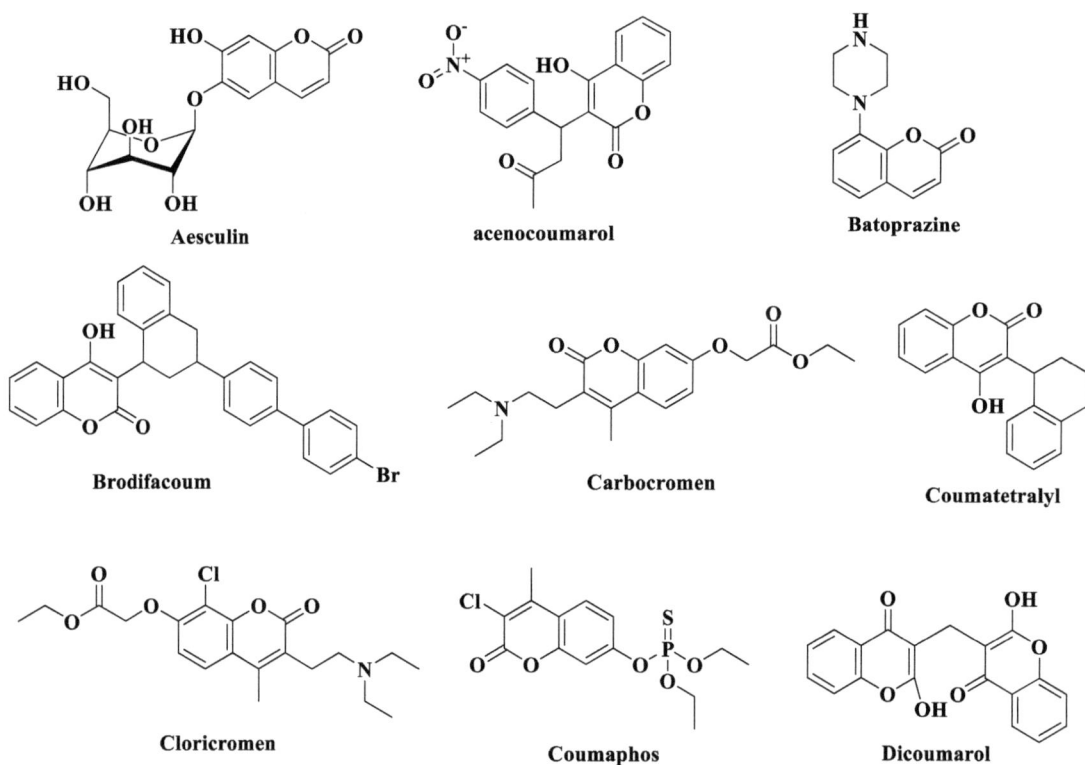

Aesculin

acenocoumarol

Batoprazine

Brodifacoum

Carbocromen

Coumatetralyl

Cloricromen

Coumaphos

Dicoumarol

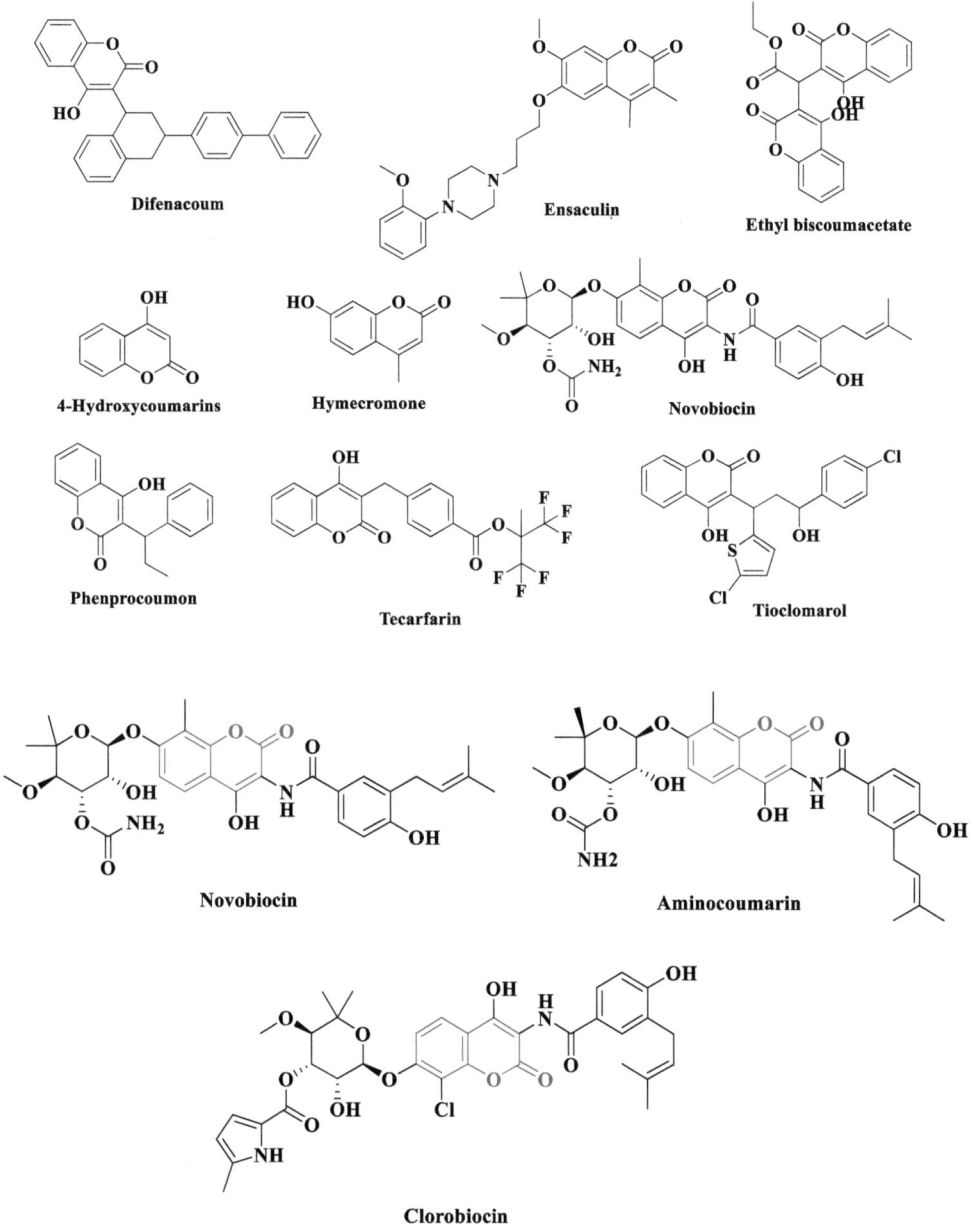

**Fig. (12).** Coumarin-based active pharmaceutical drugs used in the treatment of various diseases.

## Antibacterial Agents

Based on bacterial infections and growth, it is essential to develop antibiotics to minimise bacterial infections. The development of coumarin-based antibacterial agents is a significant area of interest because of their great activity and stability. Recent reports of coumarin-pyrazoline derivatives **E1 (a-e)** (Fig. **13**) synthesised and studied in-vitro antibacterial activity against the *Staphylococcus aureus, Escherichia coli 1411, Escherichia coli SM1411* by *Asha et al.* [58] and all synthesised compound exhibits good antibacterial activity with MIC: 14 µg/mL. Compared with reference sample D-cycloserine, E1-a shows more activity (14 µg/mL). SAR studies revealed that substitutions with methyl, hydroxy, and methoxy groups on aromatic rings favour antibacterial activities. *Singh et al.* designed and synthesised monocarbonyl curcumin-coumarin derivatives **E2 (a-d)** (Fig. **13**) and screened their biological activity against the *S. aureus* and *E. faecalis* (Gram-positive) and *P. aeruginosa* and *E. coli* (Gram-negative) strains [59]. The results revealed that Compound **E2-a** (Fig. **13**) MIC: 12.5 µg/m shown intense antibacterial activity against the *P. aeruginosa*. SAR studies reveal that methoxy substitutions on the aromatic ring-containing curcumin-coumarin derivatives exhibit the most potent antibacterial nature. Lopez *et al.* developed a 4-substituted 1,2,3-triazole-coumarin hybrids **E3 (a-e)** (Fig. **13**) and evaluated their biological activity [60]. All designed molecules are screened for their *in-vitro* antibacterial activity against the Gram-positive *Enterococcus faecalis* with MIC: 12.5 µg/mL. Among all developed compounds, **E3-b** (Fig. **13**) containing 2-Ph-OMe with triazole moiety and -OCH$_2$ linker had a good antibacterial impact on the bacterial strain with MIC: 12.5 µg/mL against *Enterococcus faecalis* and chloramphenicol as a reference drug. A simple coumarin hybrid E4 with different substitutions at R1 and R2 exhibits great *in vitro* antibacterial activity against the different bacterial strains such as *Escherichia coli, Staphylococcus aureus, Streptococcus agalactiae*, and *Flavobacterium cloumnare*. Among all these, **E4-a** (MIC: 2 µM) and **E4-b** (Fig. **13**) (MIC: 4 µM) confirmed that substations at R1 and R2 positions exhibit potential antibacterial action and which are similar in their mechanism of action when compared to the standard compound Enrofloxacin (MIC: µM) [61]. *Liu et al.* designed and synthesised coumarin-pyrazole carboxamide hybrids **E5** (Fig. **13**), and all synthesised compounds exhibited potent antibacterial activity against *E. coli* [62]. Hybrid **E5-a** (MIC: 0.25mg/L) exhibits the most potent inhibitor against *E. coli*. It exhibited a 16-fold increase in inhibition of bacterial activity when compared to Novobiocon (MIC: 4 mg/mL) and double folds high inhibitory activity than Ciprofloxacin (MIC; 0.5 mg/mL). SAR studies reveal that R1, R2, and R4 positions with different substitutions are more favourable for the antibacterial activities, and substitutions with Cl atom and carboxylic moieties are most active against the *E. coli,* and Cl and -COOEt Substitutions at R3 and R4 positions play a key role against the

*Salmenolle stains*. This study reveals that coumarin containing pyrazole carboxamide derivatives are of a great impact on antibacterial research. Green synthesis of bis-coumarin derivatives **E6** (Fig. **13**) was developed by *Chougala et al.* [63] and revealed moderate antibacterial activity against gram-positive and gram-negative bacteria. Compound **E6-b** (MIC: 3.25 µg/mL) substitution of a methyl group at the C7 position of coumarin moiety are preferably shown antibacterial activity against the E. faecalis, and at C6 position -Cl atom substitution exhibits antibacterial nature against the *E. Coli* and P. intermedia **E6-C** (Fig. **13**) (MIC: 1.56 µg/mL) compared with reference sample Ciprofloxacin (MIC:6.25 mg/mL). Chauhan's research group also studied thiazines containing coumarins **E7** (Fig. **13**) and demonstrated they possess *in vitro* antibacterial activity [64]. The preliminary results indicate that designed derivatives are shown potential antibacterial activity against the *E. coli* strain. **E7-a** (Fig. **13**) (MIC: 50 µg/mL) derivative indicated more potential antibacterial activity against *E. coli.* SAR study of these compounds reveals that electron-withdrawing groups exhibit good antibacterial activity in descending order as follows: 4-Cl > 3-Br > 4-F > 4-OH > 3-OPh on the aryl ring. This study helps to find new bacterial resistances.

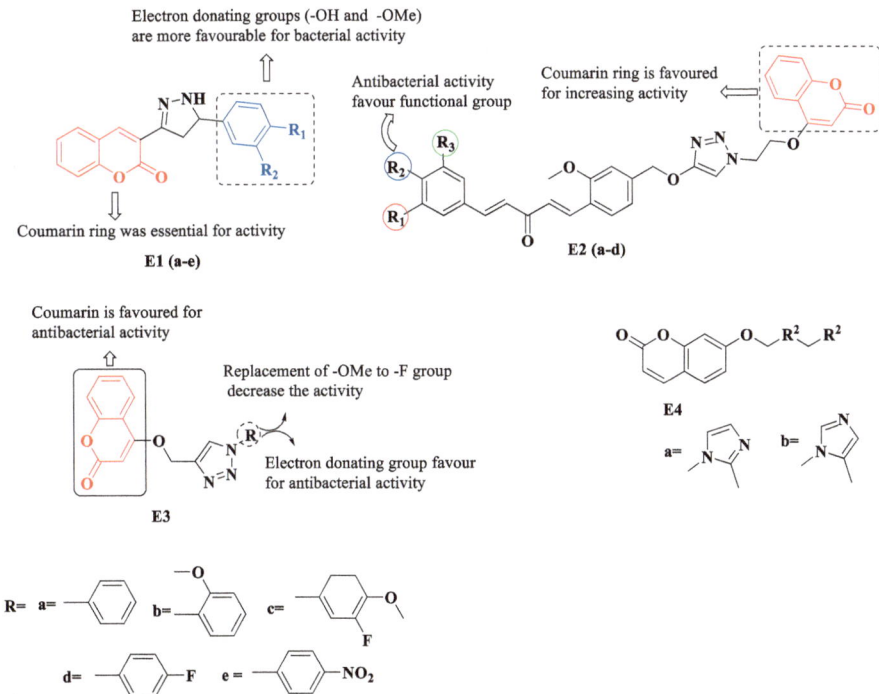

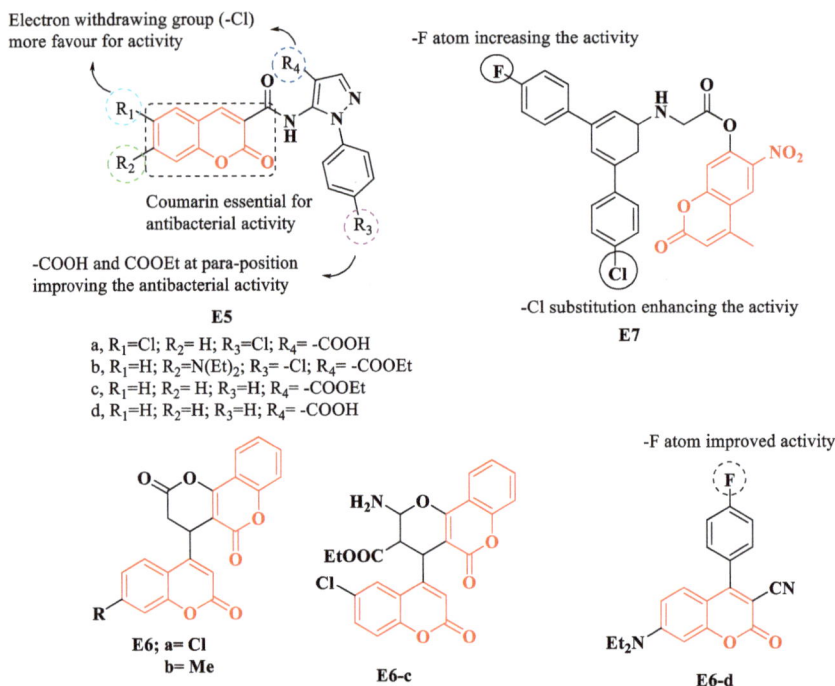

**Fig. (13).** Coumarin derivatives as potent antibacterial agents [58 - 64].

A new class of coumarin-dihydropyrimidine amide derivatives **E8** (Fig. **14**) are synthesised by *Chavan et al.,* and molecular docking studies were performed; these compounds were then screened for in-vitro antibacterial activity using the agar well diffusion method against both gram-positive and gram-negative bacteria such as *Bacillus subtilis, Staphylococcus aureus*, and *Escherichia coli, P. Aeruginosa* strains [65]. Among the series, compounds with 5,7-diCH$_3$ (MIC: 5 µg/mL) and 5,6-Benzo (MIC: 2.5 µg/mL) showed great antibacterial effects against gram-positive and negative bacteria. SAR studies show that the electron-donating group present in the coumarin moiety contributes significantly to the antibacterial activity. A series of novel nicotinonitrile-coumarin hybrids **E9** (Fig. **14**) is reported by *Sherif* and co-workers and screened for their antibacterial activity against *Escherichia coli, Klebsiella pneumonia, Pseudomonas aeruginosa* (gram-positive) and *Staphylococcus aureus, Streptococcus mutans* (gram-negative) [66]. Among all compounds, methyl-substituted derivatives (MIC: 1.9, 3.9, 3.9, 3.9, and 7.8 µg/mL) possessed the greatest potential antibacterial activity against both Gram-positive and Gram-negative bacteria compared with standard Ciprofloxacin. The in-vitro cytotoxic activity was also studied, and most of these novel hybrids performed well against human breast carcinoma cell line (MCF-7), colon cancer cell line (Caco2), and liver hepatocellular carcinoma cell line (HEPG2). All outcomes exhibit satisfactory equated cytotoxicity with Doxorubicin ($IC_{50}$: 25.17 µg/mL). A new class of coumarin-pyrazole hybrids **E10** (Fig. **14**) is synthesised using microwave irradiation and evaluated theirs *in vitro* antibacterial activity against Gram-positive bacteria such as *Bacillus subtilis and Staphylococcus aureus*, and Gram-negative bacteria such as *Escherichia coli* and *P. aeruginosa* strains. The MIC value of these newly developed compounds is compared with standard Ciprofloxacin. Among all these, 6-Cl (MIC: 0.78 µg ml$^{-1}$) and 7,8-benzo (MIC 1.562 µg ml$^{-1}$) have shown excellent bacterial effects against the gram-positive *Staphylococcus aureus* bacteria. A new variety of benzamides coupled with coumarin derivatives **E11** (Fig. **14**) is designed for the most potent antibacterial and antimicrobial activities [67]. One study was conducted in which antibacterial activity against *E. coli, S. aureus, B. subtilis,* and *P. aeruginosa* strains was observed. All compounds exhibited moderate antibacterial activity at MIC: 5 µg/mL, compared with Ciprofloxacin, whose newly developed derivatives exhibited great antibacterial activity. *In vitro* antibacterial activity study of novel uracil-coumarin-based hybrid derivatives, **E12** (Fig. **14**) exhibits improved antibacterial activity against gram-positive bacteria such as *Enterococcus faecalis* and *Staphylococcus aureus*, two Gram-negative bacteria *Pseudomonas aeruginosa* and *Escherichia coli* bacterial strains [68]. The SAR studies reveal that the substituted uracil moiety was found to be more active than the unsubstituted uracil moiety and electron-donating groups influence the inhibition potential ($F=Cl>Br>T>NO_2>CH_3>H$), and the potency decreases when the length of the chain increases. A recent study of microwave synthesis of novel triazine indole coumarin derivative **E13** (Fig. **14**) was designed and synthesized by *Sumitra N. Mangasuli* [69]. Synthesized compound exhibits antibacterial activity against *S. aureus* (MIC: 0.125 µg/mL), *B. subtilis* (MIC of 0.25 µg/mL), *E. coli* and *P. aeruginosa* (0.5 µg/mL) [67]. Green synthesis approach of coumarin-based thiazoles **E14** (Fig. **14**) is synthesized and screened their cytotoxic evolution by *Srikanth et al.* Synthesized compounds were further studied for their *in vitro* antibacterial activities against *Staphylococcus aureus* gram-positive bacterium [70]. Among all compounds, the **-Cl** substituted hybrid (MIC: 3µl/mL) exhibits significant antibacterial activity against the *S. aureus*, when compared to the standard drug (Novobiocin).

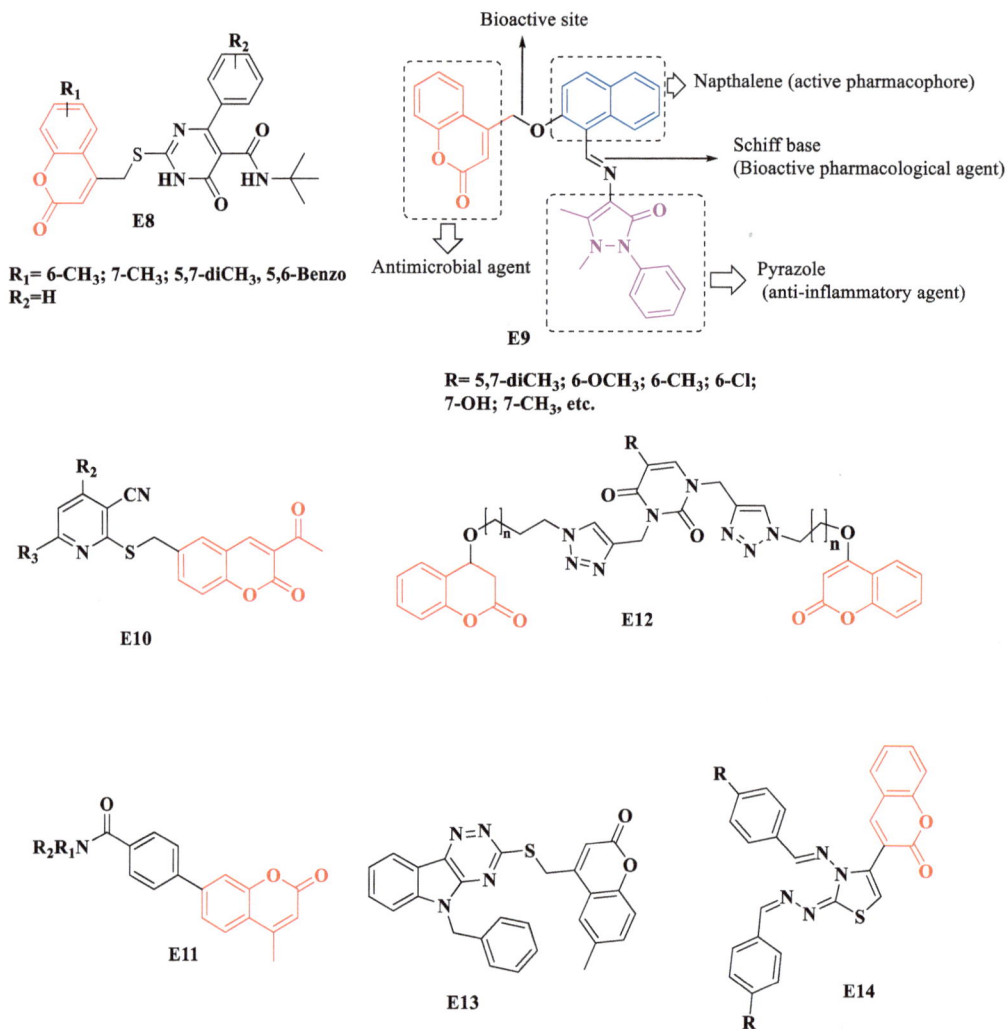

R₁= 6-CH₃; 7-CH₃; 5,7-diCH₃, 5,6-Benzo
R₂=H

R= 5,7-diCH₃; 6-OCH₃; 6-CH₃; 6-Cl;
7-OH; 7-CH₃, etc.

**Fig. (14).** Coumarin hybrids as antibacterial agents [65 - 70].

## Antiviral Activity

Coumarins possess broad antiviral activity with a different mechanism of action and its effects on viruses with their specific biological activity. Coumarins with various substitutions have been reported as a tremendous source of antiviral activity for many years, and these compounds are highly sought after by researchers looking to identify novel antiviral agents. If we look back, coumarin-derived compounds are very active in killing various viruses such as HIV, Dengue, influenza, Chikungunya, and hepatitis.

A recent report by Liu *et al.* designed and synthesized a bioactive novel prenylated coumarins **F1** (Fig. **15**) [71]. All synthesized compounds are screened for biological activity and their anti-HIV and anti-inflammatory activities. The inhibition assay of HIV-1 ($EC_{50}$) and cytotoxic activity assay were reported against C8166 cell lines according to the MTT method. In this series, compound **F1-a, F1-b, F1-C** (Fig. **15**) showed great inhibition activity with $EC_{50}$=0.29, 0.68, 0.17 µM. In 2019, Liu and co-workers were able to synthesize prenylated coumarin derivatives, for the first time, such as **F2** (Fig. **15**), from natural sources, *S., Manilkara zapota fruits* [72]. A new class of these hybrids is evaluated for potential anti-inflammatory and anti-HIV activities. A new class of these prenylated coumarins exhibits the improved anti-HIV reverse transferase effect. From this series, compounds **F2-a, F2-b**, and **F2-C** (Fig. **15**) shown more effect with $EC_{50}$: 0.12 µM.

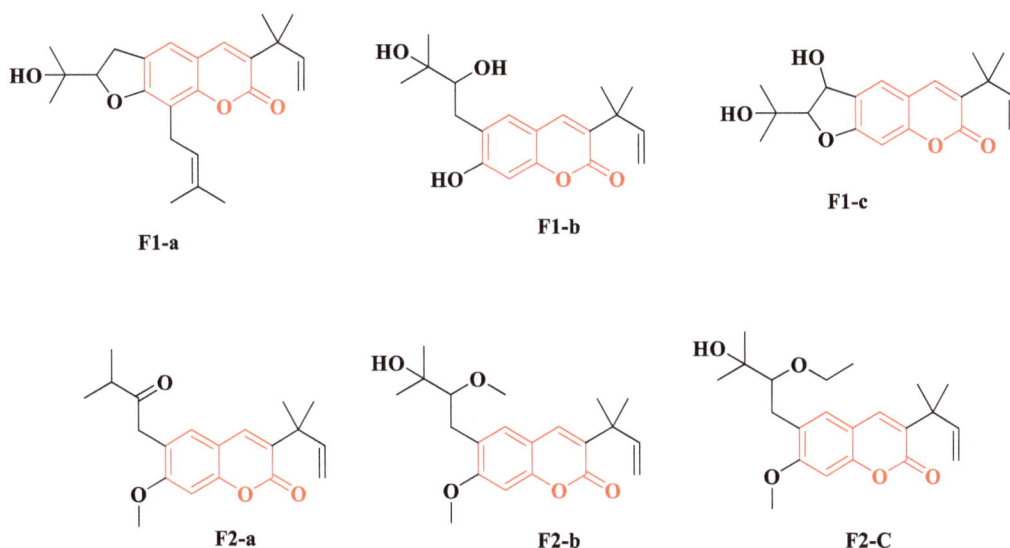

**Fig. (15).** Coumarin derivatives as antiviral hybrids [71, 72].

A new series of thiazole compounds with coumarin derivatives **F3** (Fig. **16**) is being synthesised as effective pharmacophore hybrids by *Osman et al.* [73]. All synthesised compounds are screened for their antibacterial and antiviral activity. Results indicate that methylamino substituted compounds highly inhibited the H1N1 influenza A virus ($IC_{50}$: 4.84 µM). Molecular docking studies reveal that thiazole-coumarin derivatives are the most effective and essential hybrids to develop novel antiviral drugs. Another approach of *Sreenu et al.* synthesised a bis-coumarinyl-bis-triazolothiadiazinyl ethane derivatives **F4** (Fig. **16**) and estimated their broad spectrum of viral inhibitory activity against the H1N1 virus [74]. All developed compounds have shown excellent antiviral activity with $EC_{50}=$ 20, 40 µM. A long alkyl chain containing coumarin derivatives revealed potent antiviral activity against the infectious hematopoietic necrosis virus (IHNV) [75]. Developed hybrids at $IC_{50}$ at 2.53 µM at 72h showed inhibition on IHNV glycoprotein and exhibited potential anti-IHNV effect. 2-methylimidazole with six carbon atom chain-linked coumarin hybrids **F5** (Fig. **16**) shown significantly improved antiviral activity. Coumarin derivatives having dithioacetals (Fig. **16**) exhibited antiviral activity against the anti-tobacco mosaic virus (TMV) reported by *Zhao et al.* [76]. Results of these hybrids reveal those synthesised hybrids are showed good action against the anti-TMV at $EC_{50}$: 54.2 mg/L and inactivated the viral infection. SAR study reveals that substitution of R2 position with the aliphatic group was increasing the activity.

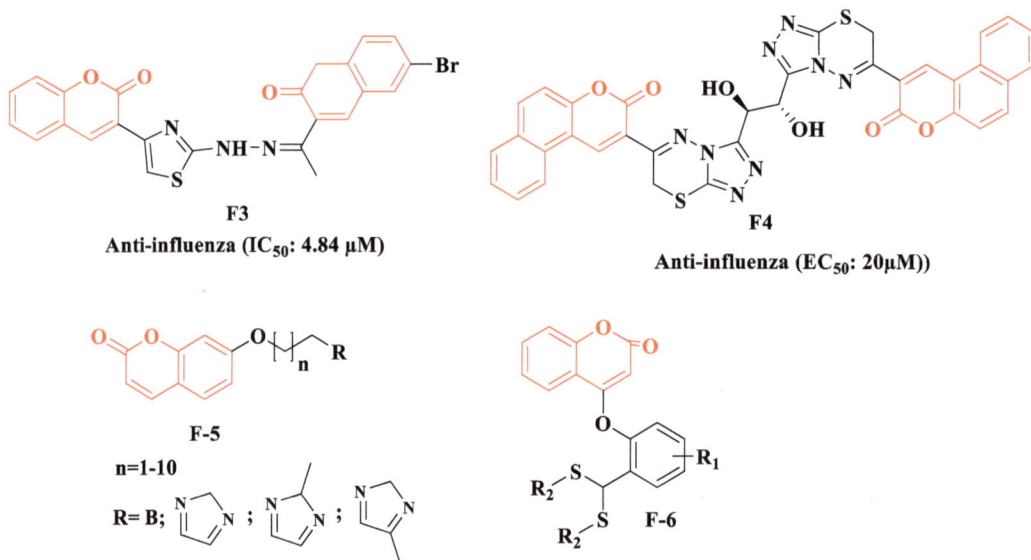

**F3**
Anti-influenza ($IC_{50}$: 4.84 µM)

**F4**
Anti-influenza ($EC_{50}$: 20µM))

**F-5**
n=1-10
R= B;

**F-6**

**Fig. (16).** benzimidazole-coumarin based antiviral agents [73 - 76].

7-(4-benzimidazole-butoxy)- **F7** (Fig. **17**) an imidazole containing coumarin derivate exhibits more potency against the *spring viraemia of carp virus* (SVCV) [77]. Compared to $IC_{50}$ values, the synthesised compound found $IC_{50}$: 0.56 mg/L exhibited more excellent antiviral activity and significantly inhibited cell death. *Tian* and co-workers have also shown that 7-(3-benzimidazole propoxy) coumarin **F8** (Fig. **17**) substantially inhibits the SVCV reproduction in fish cells and reveals that the designed compound has great antiviral activity [78]. 7-(4-(4-metyl-imidazole))-coumarin **F9** (Fig. **17**) hybrids also possess significant activity against SVCV reported by *Liu et al.* in 2019 [79]. This study states that *in vivo* inhibition of SVCV infection at 20 µg/mL using synthesised hybrids shows great antiviral activity. A new class of imidazole containing coumarin **F10** (Fig. **17**) derivatives showing excellent inhibitory activity against SVCV reproduction in host cells by activating the Nrf-2 pathway and reveals a possible way to minimise and control SVCV infection [80].

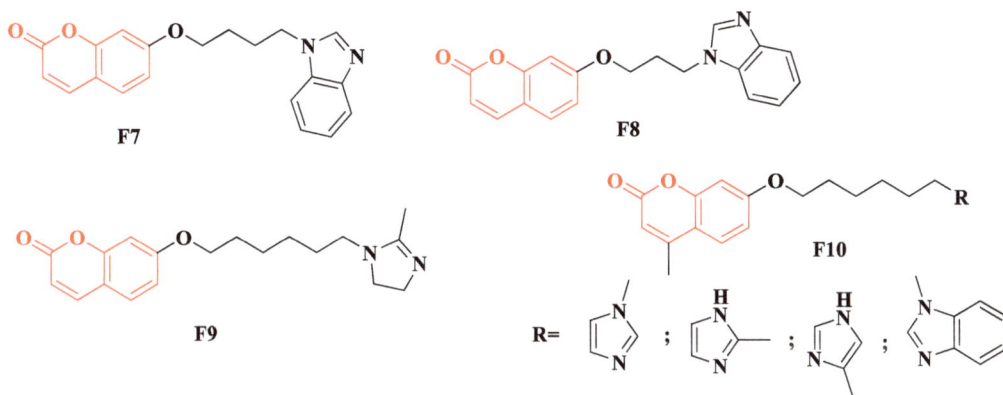

**Fig. (17).** Long alkyl chain contains coumarin derivatives as an antiviral agent [77 - 80].

## SUMMARY AND PERSPECTIVE

At present, many lethal diseases are occurring, and the entire world is fighting against different viral infections, including Nipah virus (Malaysia), Hendra virus (Australia), Hantavirus (US), Ebola virus (Africa), Zika virus (America), and the novel Coronavirus (China and the entire world). Currently, no significant drug or vaccine exists against these emerging viral diseases. This review summarises the recent developments in anti-infective agents, mainly antiviral and antibacterial agents such as 1,2,4-triazole, isatin, and coumarin-based derivatives. Moreover, we also summarised the structure-activity relationships of the reported anti-infectives. These compounds significantly influence medicinal chemistry and contain plenty of potential therapeutic applications to develop novel drugs. Many bioactive molecules substituted on leading hybrids also lead to increasing their activity. Isatin-based derivatives have become a greatly advantaged hybrid in drug developments because the isatin moiety can easily interact with receptor sites and mediate its action *via* a different mechanism of action. Coumarin hybrids also have practical importance in medicinal chemistry and the design and develop novel bioactive pharmaceuticals. Currently, this natural moiety is present in plenty of available drugs in the market. SAR results of these derivatives help understand how substituents affect the biological activity with basic Skelton. SAR studies reveal that these compounds help to treat many diseases. Many drugs are developed and currently under clinical trials, but many of these exhibit toxic side effects. Research and development on triazole, coumarin, and isatin-based compounds in the pharmaceutical industry are rapidly increasing together with their importance in treating various diseases. Moreover, the synthetic routes to develop these hybrid derivatives are easier to design and aid in discovering new potential agents. This review chapter will be valuable to encourage many researchers to design and develop sustainable, less toxic, and low-cost drugs for various diseases to decrease the mortality rate globally.

## CONSENT FOR PUBLICATION

Not applicable.

## CONFLICT OF INTEREST

The author declares no conflict of interest, financial or otherwise.

## ACKNOWLEDGEMENTS

The authors are thankful to the Department of Chemistry, GITAM University, Hyderabad, for providing all the necessary facilities.

## REFERENCES

[1]     Lou Z, Sun Y, Rao Z. Current progress in antiviral strategies. Trends Pharmacol Sci 2014; 35(2): 86-102.
        [http://dx.doi.org/10.1016/j.tips.2013.11.006] [PMID: 24439476]

[2]     Li Guangdi. Therapeutic options for the 2019 novel coronavirus (2019-nCoV). Nat Rev Drug Discov 2019; 19: 149-50.

[3]     Nathan C. Antibiotics at the crossroads. Nature 2004; 431(7011): 899-902.
        [http://dx.doi.org/10.1038/431899a] [PMID: 15496893]

[4]     Wang M, Rakesh KP, Leng J, *et al.* Amino acids/peptides conjugated heterocycles: A tool for the recent development of novel therapeutic agents. Bioorg Chem 2018; 76: 113-29.
        [http://dx.doi.org/10.1016/j.bioorg.2017.11.007] [PMID: 29169078]

[5]     Vincent JL, Rello J, Marshall J, *et al.* International study of the prevalence and outcomes of infection in intensive care units. JAMA 2009; 302(21): 2323-9.
        [http://dx.doi.org/10.1001/jama.2009.1754] [PMID: 19952319]

[6]     Cohen ML. Changing patterns of infectious disease. Nature 2000; 406(6797): 762-7.
        [http://dx.doi.org/10.1038/35021206] [PMID: 10963605]

[7]     Brown T Jr, Charlier P, Herman R, Schofield CJ, Sauvage E. Structural basis for the interaction of lactivicins with serine beta-lactamases. J Med Chem 2010; 53(15): 5890-4.
        [http://dx.doi.org/10.1021/jm100437u] [PMID: 20593835]

[8]     De Clercq E, Li G. Approved antiviral drugs over the past 50 years. Clin microbiol rev 2016; 29(3): 695-747.
        [http://dx.doi.org/10.1128/CMR.00102-15] [PMID: 27281742]

[9]     Takizawa N, Yamasaki M. Current landscape and future prospects of antiviral drugs derived from microbial products. J Antibiot (Tokyo) 2017; 71(1): 45-52.

[http://dx.doi.org/10.1038/ja.2017.115] [PMID: 29018267]

[10]    Eldehna WM, Fares M, Abdel-Aziz MM, Abdel-Aziz HA. Design, synthesis and antitubercular activity of certain nicotinic Acid hydrazides. Molecules 2015; 20(5): 8800-15.
[http://dx.doi.org/10.3390/molecules20058800] [PMID: 25988611]

[11]    Denholm JT, McBryde ES, Eisen DP, Penington JS, Chen C, Street AC. Adverse effects of isoniazid preventative therapy for latent tuberculosis infection: a prospective cohort study. Drug Healthc Patient Saf 2014; 6(6): 145-9.
[http://dx.doi.org/10.2147/DHPS.S68837] [PMID: 25364275]

[12]    Fan YL, Ke X, Liu M. Coumarin-triazole hybrids and their biological activities. J Heterocycl Chem 2018; 55: 791-802.
[http://dx.doi.org/10.1002/jhet.3112]

[13]    Zhou C-H, Wang Y. Recent researches in triazole compounds as medicinal drugs. Curr Med Chem 2012; 19(2): 239-80.
[http://dx.doi.org/10.2174/092986712803414213] [PMID: 22320301]

[14]    Pokuri S, Singla RK, Bhat VG, Shenoy GG. Insights on the antioxidant potential of 1, 2, 4-triazoles: synthesis, screening & QSAR studies. Curr Drug Metab 2014; 15(4): 389-97.
[http://dx.doi.org/10.2174/1389200215666140908101958] [PMID: 25204824]

[15]    Wu J, Ni T, Chai X, *et al.* Molecular docking, design, synthesis and antifungal activity study of novel triazole derivatives. Eur J Med Chem 2018; 143: 1840-6.
[http://dx.doi.org/10.1016/j.ejmech.2017.10.081] [PMID: 29133044]

[16]    Wang W, Wang S, Liu Y, *et al.* Novel conformationally restricted triazole derivatives with potent antifungal activity. Eur J Med Chem 2010; 45(12): 6020-6.
[http://dx.doi.org/10.1016/j.ejmech.2010.09.070] [PMID: 20950895]

[17]    Xu J, Cao Y, Zhang J, *et al.* Design, synthesis and antifungal activities of novel 1,2,4-triazole derivatives. Eur J Med Chem 2011; 46(7): 3142-8.
[http://dx.doi.org/10.1016/j.ejmech.2011.02.042] [PMID: 21420761]

[18]    Sheng C, Che X, Wang W, *et al.* Design and synthesis of novel triazole antifungal derivatives by structure-based bioisosterism. Eur J Med Chem 2011; 46(11): 5276-82.
[http://dx.doi.org/10.1016/j.ejmech.2011.03.019] [PMID: 21983332]

[19]    Zou Y, Yu S, Li R, *et al.* Synthesis, antifungal activities and molecular docking studies of novel 2-(2,4-difluorophenyl)-2-hydroxy-3-(1H-1,2,4-triazol-1-yl)propyl dithiocarbamates. Eur J Med Chem 2014; 74: 366-74.
[http://dx.doi.org/10.1016/j.ejmech.2014.01.009] [PMID: 24487187]

[20]    Li L, Ding H, Wang B, *et al.* Synthesis and evaluation of novel azoles as potent antifungal agents. Bioorg Med Chem Lett 2014; 24(1): 192-4.
[http://dx.doi.org/10.1016/j.bmcl.2013.11.037] [PMID: 24332489]

[21]    Cao X, Sun Z, Cao Y, *et al.* Design, synthesis, and structure-activity relationship studies of novel fused heterocycles-linked triazoles with good activity and water solubility. J Med Chem 2014; 57(9): 3687-706.
[http://dx.doi.org/10.1021/jm4016284] [PMID: 24564525]

[22]    Shrestha SK, Garzan A, Garneau-Tsodikova S. Novel alkylated azoles as potent antifungals. Eur J Med Chem 2017; 133: 309-18.
[http://dx.doi.org/10.1016/j.ejmech.2017.03.075] [PMID: 28395217]

[23]    Zhang Y, Tangadanchu VKR, Bheemanaboina RRY, Cheng Y, Zhou CH. Novel carbazole-triazole conjugates as DNA-targeting membrane active potentiators against clinical isolated fungi. Eur J Med Chem 2018; 155: 579-89.
[http://dx.doi.org/10.1016/j.ejmech.2018.06.022] [PMID: 29913383]

[24]    Lin GS, Duan WG, Yang LX, Huang M, Lei FH. Synthesis and antifungal activity of novel myrtenal-

based 4-methyl-1,2,4-triazole-thioethers. Molecules 2017; 22(2): 1-10.
[http://dx.doi.org/10.3390/molecules22020193] [PMID: 28125042]

[25]    Jin R-Y, Zeng C-Y, Liang XH, *et al.* Design, synthesis, biological activities and DFT calculation of novel 1,2,4-triazole Schiff base derivatives. Bioorg Chem 2018; 80: 253-60.
[http://dx.doi.org/10.1016/j.bioorg.2018.06.030] [PMID: 29966871]

[26]    Zoumpoulakis P, Camoutsis Ch, Pairas G, *et al.* Synthesis of novel sulfonamide-1,2,4-triazoles, 1,3,4-thiadiazoles and 1,3,4-oxadiazoles, as potential antibacterial and antifungal agents. Biological evaluation and conformational analysis studies. Bioorg Med Chem 2012; 20(4): 1569-83.
[http://dx.doi.org/10.1016/j.bmc.2011.12.031] [PMID: 22264752]

[27]    Tang R, Jin L, Mou C, *et al.* Synthesis, antifungal and antibacterial activity for novel amide derivatives containing a triazole moiety. Chem Cent J 2013; 7(1): 30.
[http://dx.doi.org/10.1186/1752-153X-7-30] [PMID: 23402603]

[28]    Wang Y, Damu GLV, Lv JS, Geng RX, Yang DC, Zhou CH. Design, synthesis and evaluation of clinafloxacin triazole hybrids as a new type of antibacterial and antifungal agents. Bioorg Med Chem Lett 2012; 22(17): 5363-6.
[http://dx.doi.org/10.1016/j.bmcl.2012.07.064] [PMID: 22884108]

[29]    Plech T, Kaproń B, Paneth A, *et al.* Search for factors affecting antibacterial activity and toxicity of 1,2,4-triazole-ciprofloxacin hybrids. Eur J Med Chem 2015; 97: 94-103.
[http://dx.doi.org/10.1016/j.ejmech.2015.04.058] [PMID: 25951434]

[30]    Mermer A, Faiz O, Demirbas A, Demirbas N, Alagumuthu M, Arumugam S. Piperazine-azol--fluoroquinolone hybrids: Conventional and microwave irradiated synthesis, biological activity screening and molecular docking studies. Bioorg Chem 2019; 85: 308-18.
[http://dx.doi.org/10.1016/j.bioorg.2019.01.009] [PMID: 30654222]

[31]    Gao LZ, Xie YS, Li T, Huang WL, Hu GQ. Synthesis and antibacterial activity of novel [1,2,4]triazolo[3,4-h][1,8]naphthyridine-7-carboxylic acid derivatives. Chin Chem Lett 2015; 26: 149-51.
[http://dx.doi.org/10.1016/j.cclet.2014.09.017]

[32]    Mohamed NG, Sheha MM, Hassan HY, Abdel-Hafez LJM, Omar FA. Synthesis, antimicrobial activity and molecular modeling study of 3-(5-amino-(2H)-1,2,4-triazol-3-yl]-naphthyridinones as potential DNA-gyrase inhibitors. Bioorg Chem 2018; 81: 599-611.
[http://dx.doi.org/10.1016/j.bioorg.2018.08.031] [PMID: 30248511]

[33]    Reddy CS, Rao LS, Sunitha B, Nagaraj A. Synthesis and antibacterial activity of N-substitute--[1,2,4]triazoles and 1,2,4-triazole[3,4-b][1,3,4]thiadiazines. Indian J Chem 2015; 54B: 1283-9.

[34]    Abu-Hashem AA, Hussein HAR, Abu-zied KM. Synthesis of novel 1,2,4- triazolopyrimidines and their evaluation as antimicrobial agents. Med Chem Res 2017; 26: 120-30.
[http://dx.doi.org/10.1007/s00044-016-1733-5]

[35]    Fan Z, Shi J, Luo N, Ding M, Bao X. Synthesis, crystal structure, and agricultural antimicrobial evaluation of novel quinazoline thioether derivatives incorporating the 1,2,4-triazolo[4,3□a]pyridine moiety. J Agric Food Chem 2019; 67(42): 11598-606.
[http://dx.doi.org/10.1021/acs.jafc.9b04733] [PMID: 31560195]

[36]    Cui P, Li X, Zhu M, Wang B, Liu J, Chen H. Design, synthesis and antimicrobial activities of thiouracil derivatives containing triazolo-thiadiazole as SecA inhibitors. Eur J Med Chem 2017; 127: 159-65.
[http://dx.doi.org/10.1016/j.ejmech.2016.12.053] [PMID: 28039774]

[37]    Yang L, Bao XP. Synthesis of novel 1,2,4-triazole derivatives containing the quinazolinylpiperidinyl moiety and N-(substituted phenyl)acetamide group as efficient bactericides against the phytopathogenic bacterium Xanthomonas oryzae pv. oryzae. RSC Advances 2017; 7: 34005-11.
[http://dx.doi.org/10.1039/C7RA04819J]

[38]    Cui J, Jin J, Chaudhary AS, *et al.* Design, synthesis and evaluation of triazole-pyrimidine analogues as SecA inhibitors. ChemMedChem 2016; 11(1): 43-56.
[http://dx.doi.org/10.1002/cmdc.201500447] [PMID: 26607404]

[39]    Zhang Y, Tangadanchu VKR, Cheng Y, Yang R-G, Lin J-M, Zhou C-H. Potential antimicrobial isopropanol-conjugated carbazole azoles as dual targeting inhibitors of Enterococcus faecalis. ACS Med Chem Lett 2018; 9(3): 244-9.
[http://dx.doi.org/10.1021/acsmedchemlett.7b00514] [PMID: 29541368]

[40]    Yin BT, Yan CY, Peng XM, *et al.* Synthesis and biological evaluation of α-triazolyl chalcones as a new type of potential antimicrobial agents and their interaction with calf thymus DNA and human serum albumin. Eur J Med Chem 2014; 71: 148-59.
[http://dx.doi.org/10.1016/j.ejmech.2013.11.003] [PMID: 24291568]

[41]    Goma'a HAM, Ghaly MA, Abou-zeid LA, Badria FA, Shehata IA, El-Kerdawy MM. Synthesis, biological evaluation and *in silico* studies of 1,2,4-triazole and 1,3,4-thiadiazole derivatives as antiherpetic agents. ChemistrySelect 2019; 4: 6421-8.
[http://dx.doi.org/10.1002/slct.201900814]

[42]    Kumar Biswas B, Malpani YR, Ha N, *et al.* Enterovirus inhibitory activity of C-8-tert-butyl substituted 4-aryl-6,7,8,9-tetrahydrobenzo[4,5]thieno[3,2-e][1,2,4]triazolo[4,3-a]pyrimidin-5(4H)-ones. Bioorg Med Chem Lett 2017; 27(15): 3582-5.
[http://dx.doi.org/10.1016/j.bmcl.2017.05.030] [PMID: 28587824]

[43]    El-Zahabi HSA. Synthesis, characterisation, and biological evaluation of some novel quinoxaline derivatives as antiviral agents. Arch Pharm Chem Life Sci 2017; 350: e1700028.
[http://dx.doi.org/10.1002/ardp.201700028]

[44]    Zaher NH, Mostafa MI, Altaher AY. Design, synthesis and molecular docking of novel triazole derivatives as potential CoV helicase inhibitors. Acta Pharm 2020; 70(2): 145-59.
[http://dx.doi.org/10.2478/acph-2020-0024] [PMID: 31955138]

[45]    Wang Z, Yu Z, Kang D, *et al.* Design, synthesis and biological evaluation of novel acetamide-substituted doravirine and its prodrugs as potent HIV-1 NNRTIs. Bioorg Med Chem 2019; 27(3): 447-56.
[http://dx.doi.org/10.1016/j.bmc.2018.12.039] [PMID: 30606670]

[46]    Mishra P, Kumar A, Mamidi P, *et al.* Inhibition of Chikungunya Virus Replication by 1-[(--Methylbenzimidazol-1-yl) Methyl]-2-Oxo-Indolin-3-ylidene] Amino] Thiourea(MBZM-N-IBT). Sci Rep 2016; 6: 20122.
[http://dx.doi.org/10.1038/srep20122] [PMID: 26843462]

[47]    N Nisha, R Tran, D Yang, *et al.* Cu(I)Cl-promoted synthesis of novel N-alkylated isatin analogs with an extension toward isatin-4-aminoquinoline conjugates: *in vitro* analysis against *Trichomonas vaginalis*. Med Chem Res 2014; 23: 4570-8.

[48]    Kumar K, Liu N, Yang D, *et al.* Synthesis and antiprotozoal activity of mono- and bis-uracil isatin conjugates against the human pathogen Trichomonas vaginalis. Bioorg Med Chem 2015; 23(16): 5190-7.
[http://dx.doi.org/10.1016/j.bmc.2015.04.075] [PMID: 25999204]

[49]    Abdulhamid Ganim Ramadan M, Cengiz Baloglu M, Celik Altunoglu Y, *et al.* Evaluation of Biological Activity of 5-Fluoro-Isatin Thiosemicarbazone Derivatives. J Nanostruct 2020; 10(3): 509-17.

[50]    Bhagat K, Bhagat J, Gupta MK, *et al.* Design, synthesis, antimicrobial evaluation, and molecular modeling studies of novel indolinedione– coumarin molecular hybrids. ACS Omega 2019; 4: 8720-30.

[51]    Almutairi MS, Zakaria AS, Ignasius PP, Al-Wabli RI, Joe IH, Attia MI. Synthesis, spectroscopic investigations, DFT studies, molecular docking and antimicrobial potential of certain new indole-isatin molecular hybrids: E. and theoretical approaches. J Mol Struct 2018; 1153: 333-45.

[http://dx.doi.org/10.1016/j.molstruc.2017.10.025]

[52]    Wang R, Yin X, Zhang Y, Yan W. Design, synthesis and antimicrobial evaluation of propylene-tethered ciprofloxacin-isatin hybrids. Eur J Med Chem 2018; 156: 580-6.
        [http://dx.doi.org/10.1016/j.ejmech.2018.07.025] [PMID: 30025351]

[53]    X Jin, Y Xu, X Chen, et al . Design, synthesis and *in vitro* anti-microbial evaluation of ethylene/propylene-1h-1,2,3-triazole-4-methylene-tethered isatin-coumarin hybrids Curr Top Med Chem 2017; 17: 3213.

[54]    Guo H. Design, synthesis and antibacterial evaluation of propylene-tethered 8-methoxyl ciprofloxacin-isatin hybrids. J Chem 2018; 55: 2434-40.

[55]    Gao F, Chen Z, Ma L, Fan Y, Chen L, Lu G. Synthesis and biological evaluation of moxifloxacin-acetyl-1,2,3-1H-triazole-methylene-isatin hybrids as potential anti-tubercular agents against both drug-susceptible and drug-resistant Mycobacterium tuberculosis strains. Eur J Med Chem 2019; 180: 648-55.
        [http://dx.doi.org/10.1016/j.ejmech.2019.07.057] [PMID: 31352245]

[56]    Gao F, Wang T, Gao M, *et al.* Benzofuran-isatin-imine hybrids tethered *via* different length alkyl linkers: Design, synthesis and *in vitro* evaluation of anti-tubercular and anti-bacterial activities as well as cytotoxicity. Eur J Med Chem 2019; 165: 323-31.
        [http://dx.doi.org/10.1016/j.ejmech.2019.01.042] [PMID: 30690301]

[57]    Stefanachi A, Leonetti F, Pisani L, Catto M, Carotti A. Coumarin: a natural, privileged and versatile scaffold for bioactive compounds. Molecules 2018; 23(2): E250.
        [http://dx.doi.org/10.3390/molecules23020250] [PMID: 29382051]

[58]    Chate AV, Redlawar AA, Bondle GM, Sarkate AP, Tiwaric SV, Lokwani DK. A new efficient domino approach for the synthesis of coumarin-pyrazolines as antimicrobial agents targeting bacterial D-alanine- D-alanine ligase. New J Chem 2019; 43: 9002-11.
        [http://dx.doi.org/10.1039/C9NJ00703B]

[59]    Singh A, Singh JV, Rana A, *et al.* Monocarbonyl curcumin-based molecular hybrids as potent antibacterial agents. ACS Omega 2019; 4(7): 11673-84.
        [http://dx.doi.org/10.1021/acsomega.9b01109] [PMID: 31460274]

[60]    Lopez-Rojas P, Janeczko M, Kubinski K, Amesty A, Masłyk M. A. Estevez- Braun, Synthesis and antimicrobial activity of 4-substituted 1,2,3-triazolecoumarin derivatives. Molecules 2018; 23: 199-217.
        [http://dx.doi.org/10.3390/molecules23010199]

[61]    Hu Y, Shen Y, Wu X, Tu X, Wang GX. Synthesis and biological evaluation of coumarin derivatives containing imidazole skeleton as potential antibacterial agents. Eur J Med Chem 2018; 143: 958-69.
        [http://dx.doi.org/10.1016/j.ejmech.2017.11.100] [PMID: 29232586]

[62]    Liu H, Ren ZL, Wang W, *et al.* Novel coumarin-pyrazole carboxamide derivatives as potential topoisomerase II inhibitors: Design, synthesis and antibacterial activity. Eur J Med Chem 2018; 157: 81-7.
        [http://dx.doi.org/10.1016/j.ejmech.2018.07.059] [PMID: 30075404]

[63]    Chougala BM, Samundeeswari S, Holiyachi M, *et al.* Joshi, V.A. Sunagar, Green, unexpected synthesis of bis-coumarin derivatives as potent antibacterial and anti-inflammatory agents. Eur J Med Chem 2018; 157: 81-7.

[64]    Chauhan NB, Patel NB, Patel VM, Mistry BM. Synthesis and biological evaluation of coumarin clubbed thiazines scaffolds as antimicrobial and antioxidant. Med Chem Res 2017; 27: 2141-9.
        [http://dx.doi.org/10.1007/s00044-018-2222-9]

[65]    Chavan RR, Hosamani KM, Kulkarni BD, Joshi SD. Molecular docking studies and facile synthesis of most potent biologically active N-tert-butyl-4-(4-substituted phenyl)-2-((substituted-2-o-o-2H-chromen-4-yl)methylthio)-6-oxo-1,6-dihydropyrimidine-5-carboxamide hybrids: An approach

for microwave-assisted syntheses and biological evaluation. Bioorg Chem 2018; 78: 185-94.
[http://dx.doi.org/10.1016/j.bioorg.2018.03.007] [PMID: 29579642]

[66]    Sherif MH. Sanad & Ahmed E. M. Mekky. Synthesis, in-vitro antibacterial and anticancer screening of novel nicotinonitrile-coumarin hybrids utilising piperazine citrate. Synth Commun 2020; 50(10): 1468-85.
[http://dx.doi.org/10.1080/00397911.2020.1743318]

[67]    Joy MN, Bakulev VA, Bodke YD, Telkar S. Synthesis of coumarins coupled with benzamides as potent antimicrobial agents. Pharm Chem J 2020; 54(6): 604-20.
[http://dx.doi.org/10.1007/s11094-020-02245-4]

[68]    Sanduja M, Gupta J, Singh H, Pagare PP, Rana A. Uracil-coumarin based hybrid molecules as potent anticancer and antibacterial agents. J Saudi Chem Soc 2019; 24: 251-66.
[http://dx.doi.org/10.1016/j.jscs.2019.12.001]

[69]    Mangasuli SN. Microwave Assisted Synthesis and Biological activity of a novel Triazino indole-Coumarin hybrid: Crystal structure, Hirshfeld surface analysis and DFT calculations. Chemical Data Collections 2020; p. 100503.

[70]    Mamidala S, Peddi SR, Aravilli RK, Jilloju PC, Manga PV, Vedula PRR. Microwave irradiated one pot, three component synthesis of a new series of hybrid coumarin based thiazoles: antibacterial evaluation and molecular docking studies. J Mol Struct 2020; 1225: 129114.

[71]    Liu YP, Yan G, Xie YT, *et al.* Bioactive prenylated coumarins as potential anti-inflammatory and anti-HIV agents from Clausena lenis. Bioorg Chem 2020; 97: 103699.
[http://dx.doi.org/10.1016/j.bioorg.2020.103699] [PMID: 32146173]

[72]    Liu YP, Yan G, Guo JM, *et al.* Prenylated Coumarins from the Fruits of *Manilkara zapota* with Potential Anti-inflammatory Effects and Anti-HIV Activities. J Agric Food Chem 2019; 67(43): 11942-7.
[http://dx.doi.org/10.1021/acs.jafc.9b04326] [PMID: 31622090]

[73]    Osman H, Yusufzai SK, Khan MS, *et al.* New thiazolyl-coumarin hybrids: Design, synthesis, characterisation, X-ray crystal structure, antibacterial and antiviral evaluation. J Mol Struct 2018; 1166: 147-54.
[http://dx.doi.org/10.1016/j.molstruc.2018.04.031]

[74]    Pavurala S, Vaarla K, Kesharwani R, Naesens L, Liekens S, Vedula RR. Bis coumarinyl bis triazolothiadiazinyl ethane derivatives: Synthesis, antiviral activity evaluation, and molecular docking studies. Synth Commun 2018; 48(12): 1494-503.
[http://dx.doi.org/10.1080/00397911.2018.1455871]

[75]    Hu Y, Chen W, Shen Y, Zhu B, Wang G-X. Synthesis and antiviral activity of coumarin derivatives against infectious hematopoietic necrosis virus. Bioorg Med Chem Lett 2019; 29(14): 1749-55.
[http://dx.doi.org/10.1016/j.bmcl.2019.05.019] [PMID: 31104994]

[76]    Zhao L, Zhang J, Liu T, *et al.* Design, synthesis, and antiviral activities of coumarin derivatives containing dithioacetal structures. J Agric Food Chem 2020; 68(4): 975-81.
[http://dx.doi.org/10.1021/acs.jafc.9b06861] [PMID: 31891504]

[77]    Shen Y-F, Liu L, Feng C-Z, *et al.* Synthesis and antiviral activity of a new coumarin derivative against spring viraemia of carp virus. Fish Shellfish Immunol 2018; 81: 57-66.
[http://dx.doi.org/10.1016/j.fsi.2018.07.005] [PMID: 29981474]

[78]    Qiu T-X, Song D-W, Shan L-P, Liu G-L, Liu L. Potential prospect of a therapeutic agent against spring viraemia of carp virus in aquaculture. Aquaculture 2019; 515: 734558.

[79]    Liu G, Wang C, Wang H, *et al.* Antiviral efficiency of a coumarin derivative on spring viremia of carp virus *in vivo*. Virus Res 2019; 268: 11-7.
[http://dx.doi.org/10.1016/j.virusres.2019.05.007] [PMID: 31095989]

[80] Liu L, Hu Y, Shen Y-F, Wang G-X, Zhu B. Evaluation on antiviral activity of coumarin derivatives against spring viraemia of carp virus in epithelioma papulosum cyprini cells. Antiviral Res 2017; 144: 173-85.
[http://dx.doi.org/10.1016/j.antiviral.2017.06.007] [PMID: 28624462]

---

# SUBJECT INDEX

## A

Abortive infection 61
Acetyl transferase 25
Acid(s) 28, 36, 40, 60, 61, 69, 72, 120, 122, 125, 126, 127, 128
  caffeic 128
  carboxylic 36
  fatty 126, 127
  Kojic 125
  nucleic 60, 61, 69
  phenolic 120
  phosphoric 28
  Rosmarinic 120
  salicylic 120, 122
  stomach 72
  ursolic 40, 120
*Acinetobacter* 5, 76, 112, 149
  *baumannii* 5, 76, 112
  *haemolyticus* 149
Acquired immunodeficiency syndrome 140
Activity 4, 29, 30, 31, 34, 36, 37, 88, 121, 123, 129, 142, 144, 146, 148, 149, 151, 152, 166, 167
  antidepressant 142
  bactericidal 4, 88, 129
  cytochrome P450-dependent enzyme 142
  gyrase 121
  metabolic 129
  protease 123
Acyl 25, 116, 122, 124, 127, 129
  carrier protein 25
  homoserine lactones (AHLs) 116, 122, 124, 127, 129
ADP-heptose synthase 27
Agents 2, 24, 29, 53, 75, 89, 112, 119, 140
  antioxidant 29
  bacteriostatic 140
  chemotherapeutic 112
  prophylactic 53, 75
Alamin adenosyl transferase 26
*Allium sativum* 122

Anthranilateisomerase 25
Antibacterial therapy 50
Antibiotic 114, 116
  biosynthesis 116
  resistant pathogens 114
Anti-infecting agents 139
Anti-inflammatory activities 165
Antimicrobial 75, 111, 112, 113, 119, 139, 140, 149, 150, 155, 158, 163
  activities 149, 150, 155, 163
  agents 75, 139, 140, 158
  resistance 111, 112, 113, 119
Antitubercular agents 156
Antiviral activity 142, 151, 164, 165, 166
Apoptosis 38
Aqueous extract propolis (AEP) 33
*Aspergillus* 144, 146, 149
  *flavus* 146
  *fumigatus* 144, 149
Assay 4, 27, 28, 165
  cytotoxic activity 165
  enzyme-linked immunosorbent 4, 27
  immune 28
ATP-dependent Clp protease 27
Autoimmune reactions 8

## B

*Bacillus subtilis* 149, 155, 162
Bacteria 51, 52, 55, 56, 60, 61, 62, 64, 65, 71, 72, 74, 81, 86, 94, 111, 112, 127, 149
  phytopathogenic 149
  planktonic 111
Bacterial autolysis 52
*B. cepacia* complex (BCC) 86
Bioinformatics 3, 4
  programs 4
  tools 3
Biosynthesis 24, 26, 124, 125, 142
  ergosterol 142
  inhibited violacein 125
  peptidoglycan 24

# Z

www.ingramcontent.com/pod-product-compliance
Lightning Source LLC
Chambersburg PA
CBHW041702210326
41598CB00007B/508